SO-BJL-290

PRACTITIONER'S GUIDE TO
DYNAMIC ASSESSMENT

donated by
e urall. h... , Psy.D.
(GSAPP, 1977)

The Guilford School Practitioner Series

EDITORS

STEPHEN N. ELLIOTT, Ph.D.
University of Wisconsin—Madison

JOSEPH C. WITT, Ph.D.
Louisiana State University, Baton Rouge

PRACTITIONER'S GUIDE TO DYNAMIC ASSESSMENT

CAROL S. LIDZ, Psy.D.
Temple University

THE GUILFORD PRESS
New York   London

© 1991 The Guilford Press
A Division of Guilford Publications, Inc.
72 Spring Street, New York, NY 10012

All rights reserved

No part of this book may be reproduced, stored in a retrieval system,
or transmitted, in any form or by any means, electronic, mechanical,
photocopying, microfilming, recording, or otherwise, without written
permission from the Publisher.

Printed in the United States of America

This book is printed on acid-free paper.

Last digit is print number: 9   8   7   6   5   4   3   2   1

Library of Congress Cataloging-in-Publication Data
Lidz, Carol Schneider.
    Practitioner's guide to dynamic assessment / Carol S. Lidz.
        p.   cm. — (The Guilford school practitioner series)
    Includes bibliographical references and index.
    ISBN 0-89862-363-4 (hardcover). — ISBN 0-89862-242-5 (pbk.)
    1. Learning disabilities — Diagnosis.   2. Learning Potential
Assessment Device.   I. Title.   II. Series.
RJ496.L4L54   1991
616.85′889075 — dc20   91-13657
                                                                   CIP

This book is dedicated to
Reuven Feuerstein,
Carl Haywood,
and
Mogens Jensen,
who "mediated" dynamic assessment
into my life.

About the Author

CAROL S. LIDZ is on the faculty of the School Psychology Program of Temple University, where she coordinates the early childhood specialization and teaches assessment courses. She continues on a consultative basis with the Clinic Team of United Cerebral Palsy Association, an interdisciplinary service for Philadelphia Head Start and day care children and their families. This is her second book on dynamic assessment. The first was an edited text, bringing together the major contributors to this developing area. Dr. Lidz has worked as a school psychologist for over 25 years, and has special interests in diagnostic assessment and intervention with young children and facilitation of parent–child interaction. She received her B.A. in psychology from the University of Michigan, her M.A. in school psychology from the University of Tennessee, and her Psy.D. in school psychology from Rutgers University.

Preface

This volume, like others in this series, strives to arm the practicing educational specialist with the most up-to-date tools available to meet the needs of students experiencing learning difficulties. Unlike some of the previous volumes, this book does not directly address the content of the learner's curriculum. Diagnostic questions involving such content are best dealt with by means of the direct assessment approaches described by Shapiro (1989; see also Rosenfield, 1987), and the curriculum-based measures described in the edited volume by Shinn (1989). This book tackles an especially complex and difficult area that incorporates such ephemeral concepts as "process" and "potential." This book is about dynamic assessment.

The proponents of dynamic assessment have assumed a very difficult challenge: to address the very core and essence of teaching and learning. Practitioners of dynamic assessment are interested in how learners learn, why errors are made, and how current levels of functioning can be improved. Questions are being asked about reliability and validity that have never been asked of traditional approaches, yet that appear much more central to assessment concerns. These include the following: To what extent do assessors viewing the same performance arrive at similar conclusions and recommendations? Do the results of the assessment lead to effective classroom interventions? How useful do teachers find the assessment results?

Although models of dynamic assessment vary, most share incorporation of a test–intervene–retest format, as well as a focus on learner modifiability and on underlying metacognitive processes that facilitate learning. The role of assessor as active interventionist rather than as passive recorder is also a common ingredient. Thus, the response to the question of what is "dynamic" about dynamic assessment is threefold:

1. The assessor actively works to facilitate learning and induce active participation in the learner.
2. The assessment focuses on process rather than product—in this case, the processes of metacognition.
3. The assessment produces information about learner modifiability and the means by which change is best accomplished.

This is the fourth book that has been written on the topic of dynamic assessment. The first, Feuerstein's (1979) classic text, served as the primary catalyst to this area of assessment. The second, an edited text (Lidz, 1987a), provided a forum for many of the major researchers and procedure developers to describe their work. The third, edited by Gupta and Coxhead (1988), included contributions from a number of the European researchers who have been actively involved in development and application of dynamic assessment procedures.

The present text summarizes ongoing work and existing models of dynamic assessment, but emphasizes implications for the practitioner. Most of all, the text attempts to equip the practitioner with the basic tools for carrying out a dynamic assessment. It must be cautioned, however, that there are obvious limitations to what a written document can provide to a practitioner. Just as good clinical interviewing skills cannot be derived solely from a text, a written reference is nevertheless necessary to provide the foundation and guidelines for the applied skills. All good diagnostic assessment is partly art, and there is no substitute for expert modeling and supervision. Dynamic assessment in particular involves clinical judgment, inference, and artful interaction. The potential for computerization of this approach is quite limited. The potential for practitioners becoming bored with assessment is also limited.

This text does not prepare practitioners to administer procedures such as the Learning Potential Assessment Device (LPAD). These procedures are described and discussed, but there is a need for additional hands-on training. The reader is provided with an understanding of the generic aspects of dynamic assessment, as well as specific ideas I have developed, so that applications can be attempted.

Although dynamic assessors need to be well versed in the basic foundations of test and measurement theory, the audience for this model is broad. The model is adaptable for diagnostic specialists within the fields of school/clinical psychology, special/regular education, and speech/language pathology. I myself am a school psychologist; the information presented here no doubt reflects this point of view and experience base. However, the reader should always be asking, "How can I adapt this to my situation?" I have also been most strongly influenced by Feuerstein's approach to dynamic assessment. This model provides the most elaborate theoretical basis. Furthermore, I view Feuerstein's concept of the Mediated Learning Experience (MLE) as vital and central to the essence of the dynamic assessment interaction. However, I have used Feuerstein's model as a basis for adaptation and modification, and do not strictly follow all of the model's details. This will become clearer in what follows.

Frequently, when a new model is proposed, the implication is that all preceding models are wrong and should be discarded. Dynamic assessment is not intended as a substitute for existing approaches. Dynamic assessment is presented as a unique and important addition to the diagnostician's repertory. Dynamic assessment responds to questions that are not addressed by other procedures. When the diagnostic question concerns how students compare in current levels of performance with age or grade peers, the procedure of choice is norm-referenced. When the diagnostic question concerns the location of a student's skills or developmental accomplishments within a predetermined hierarchy, the procedure of choice is developmentally referenced. When the diagnostic question concerns the specific knowledge base the student has or has not acquired, the procedure of choice is criterion- or curriculum-referenced. When the diagnostic question concerns the responsiveness of the learner to intervention, the repertory of problem-solving processes employed or not employed, and the means by which change is best effected, the procedure of choice is dynamic. Dynamic assessment makes an important contribution to the direct assessment of the learner. Within an ecologically valid model, additional procedures need to be included to assess environmental contributions to the observed performance. None of these procedures is inherently better than another. Each is the best procedure for a particular issue, and no good practitioner relies on a single approach for all the answers. As diagnostic specialists, we need always to ask, "What do we need to know, and what will generate the appropriate information?" Assessment is a cognitive process; it is not equal to the number and nature of the assessment instruments administered.

Dynamic assessment is the "new kid on the block" of assessment procedures. Although it is (I believe) beyond infancy, it remains in the relatively early stages of development. More research is needed (when is this not the case?), but there is some good research currently available. I hope that readers will be sufficiently impressed with the potential of this approach to generate meaningful information and that this book will stimulate further research as well as commitment to training of new practitioners.

This text is divided into three sections. Part I includes a presentation, critique, and discussion of existing models of dynamic assessment; a special chapter on applications of the model to preschool populations;

and a review and discussion of research involving these models. However, research related to properties of the specific instruments discussed is covered in the chapters describing these procedures. Part II elaborates on the Mediated Learning Experience Rating Scale, an instrument I have developed; this scale derives primarily from Feuerstein's theories, but reflects my own reviews of the parent–child interaction and cognitive-developmental research as well. Part III consists of an elaboration of my proposed model of dynamic assessment, and of descriptions of a "generic" and a curriculum-referenced approach to dynamic assessment, along with case illustrations. Although each section is meant to "stand alone" in terms of its description of the measures involved, the theory base is not repeated, and the reader is referred to Part I for elaboration of Feuerstein's basic theories.

CAROL S. LIDZ

Contents

I

FOUNDATIONS OF
DYNAMIC ASSESSMENT

1

Introduction

Dynamic assessment is an approach that sounds so logical and convincing to practitioners that they often think they are already using it, when in fact they are not. What makes more sense than to say, "If you want to find out how a child learns, then teach him," or "The best link to classroom intervention is a sample intervention," or "It is more important to find out how responsive the child is to intervention than to focus on what she already knows"?* What often passes as dynamic assessment to the practitioner not specifically trained in this approach is best described as "testing limits," or in some cases, "trial or diagnostic teaching." Dynamic assessment as described in this book is neither. What, then, is it?

The terms "learning potential assessment" and "dynamic assessment" have been used interchangeably to indicate the model of assessment described in this book. Both Budoff (e.g., 1987a, 1987b) and Feuerstein have used the term "learning potential," and Feuerstein (1979) offered "dynamic assessment" in his classic text describing his procedure. "Dynamic assessment" has been selected as the term of choice for this text, since it describes the nature of the assessment procedure, rather than suggesting an examinee's outcome in a way that many find controversial and questionable. Whether it is "potential" that is revealed by the assessment is not central to understanding or acceptance of the model. To argue whether potential can be assessed will serve only as a distraction.

Dynamic assessment is typically contrasted with static assessment. This reflects the fact that dynamic assessment focuses on learning

---

*A note on the use of pronouns in this book is in order. For the most part, I have chosen to alternate between "he" and "she," rather than to use "he or she."

processes, in contrast to the traditional assessment focus on already learned *products.* When product is the outcome there is no information regarding the reason for failure or the learner's ability to achieve. There are also no guidelines or implications for intervention to connect the assessment with intervention and to make the assessment relevant for an educational setting. In the case of curriculum-based assessment, the product outcome allows awareness of the next educational step, but fails to provide information about how to get there. Even in the case when there are well-accepted teaching practices for specific objectives, there are always individuals who do not profit from such techniques. These are the individuals who are typically referred for individual assessment, and who challenge the relevance and adequacy of our prevailing assessment practices.

Dynamic assessment raises questions about our current conceptualizations of intelligence, at least as typically reflected in assessment procedures. Measures of intelligence are most often validated in terms of product-based criteria (i.e., achievement tests). Tests of learning ability typically do not yield high correlations either with traditional measures of intelligence or with their static criteria. One interpretation is to say that tests of learning ability are not measuring "intelligence." It could also be asserted that neither IQ tests nor their achievement-based criteria are valid reflections of intelligence. All that can be clearly concluded from the existing evidence is that these two phenomena are different; IQ is not learning ability. Whether either or neither is "intelligence" remains to be studied and debated. The concern here is with determination of strategies that facilitate learning within the educational setting. As assessors, we value both types of information: level of performance, as well as ability to profit from instruction and intervention. Dynamic assessment will inform us regarding the latter.

DEFINITION

Although there are variations in the interpretation of the dynamic assessment model, there are certain core criteria that tend to define this approach. First, as I have indicated in the preface, is a test–intervene–retest format. The specialist first administers a static pretest to establish a level of performance, then provides interventions to try to produce changes in the examinee, and then retests on the static test in order to assess degree and nature of change; the change is interpreted in terms of "response to instruction" or "intervention." Procedures differ considerably regarding the specifics of the pretests and posttests administered, as well as in terms of the interventions provided. There are also significant differences regarding the degree to which the processes addressed in the learner are articulated; some procedures do not discuss this at all, whereas others go to considerable length to define and describe learner processing variables.

A second definitive characteristic of a dynamic assessment is the focus on learner modifiability. "Modifiability" involves both the amount of change made by the learner in response to the interventions provided, and the learner's increased implementation of relevant metacognitive processes in problem solution. However, failure to change during the course of the assessment may reflect either the resistance of the learner or the inadequacy of the interventions. Nevertheless, this is the major outcome information of this model of assessment, in contrast to the level-of-performance information yielded by traditional static measures. It is very difficult to interpret this information, however. Ideally, learner response should be viewed as the criterion of success for the interventions provided; instead, there has been a temptation to use this information as a basis for classification, a means of presenting old problems in new guises.

There is justification for deriving conclusions regarding the intensity of intervention necessary for inducing change in the learner. This may indeed have implications for which students warrant full-time versus part-time placements — but therein also lies the trap. Dynamic assessment was never intended to offer an alternative basis either for classifying children or for placing them in special education programs. Information from these assessments may add to other information to aid in such decision making, but the intent of dynamic assessment is to improve understanding of the learner within any educational setting, as well as to inform interventions within any setting. Furthermore, there is no evidence to justify that dynamic assessment will improve either classification or placement decisions. Dynamic assessment is not a prescriptor for special education models; it is a diagnostic approach that is adaptable to any existing education practice. It is possible to conceive of gifted as well as retarded levels of performance in learners who are easily modifiable, as well as not so easily modifiable; that is, there can just as well be a student with gifted levels of performance who is low on indices of modifiability as there can be a student with deficient levels of performance who is high on such parameters. An assessment procedure will not solve the larger issues of programming, although such a procedure may provide a tool to facilitate relevant individualized programming under more or less restrictive conditions, and may empower teachers and their consultants to meet a larger number of student needs within less restrictive settings.

This leads to the third defining characteristic of dynamic assessment:

The assessment provides useful information for developing interventions. During the course of the assessment, the specialist provides a variety of interventions; some of these will lead to success on the task, whereas others will produce negative or possibly neutral responses. In procedures that do not provide predetermined interventions, there is a great deal of latitude for experimentation and for hypothesis derivation and confirmation. There is also a great deal of pressure on the assessor to analyze the learner's needs and then to devise a means of response. The assessor must also meticulously record what interventions appear to work or not to work, so that these can be discussed with the teacher and parent.

Additional information that can be derived from this approach to assessment involves the intensity of intervention required to produce change. Although there are sometimes means of operationalizing this information, such as listing number of times of presentation until mastery, this often is largely a matter of judgment. However, it is likely that independent judges could agree on gross categories of intensity, and this is certainly a testable assertion.

Thus, we can define dynamic assessment as an approach that follows a test–intervene–retest format, and that focuses on learner modifiability and on producing suggestions for interventions that appear successful in facilitating improved learner performance. Dynamic assessment also provides information regarding functional and dysfunctional metacognitive processes, as well as regarding intensity of intervention involved in producing change.

Dynamic assessment is unquestionably more time-consuming than most other approaches, especially when individually administered. Group-administrable procedures have been developed by both Feuerstein and Budoff (see Budoff, 1987b; Rand & Kaniel, 1987) that require considerably less time than individually administered approaches. These group-administered procedures provide valuable diagnostic information to the teacher, and also allow screening of students who require more individual attention. It is neither efficient nor relevant to administer a dynamic assessment to all referred students. As is true for any procedure, the approach should be selected in order to respond to specific diagnostic questions. Most dynamic procedures involve a number of "tests," which allow the specialist to control the time of administration. However, sufficient time is required to permit learning to take place; just how much time is enough is a matter of judgment. This is clearly not the procedure of choice for any quick assessment needs.

Dynamic assessment, as discussed in this book, needs to be distinguished from both testing of limits and diagnostic teaching. The model differs from testing of limits in its considerably broader scope and intent. Limit testing is still bound to static concepts, and is carried out unsystematically, within relatively brief spurts of time. Typically, an assessor will provide extensions of time on timed tests, or vary vocabulary on comprehension tests, or simplify the number of stimuli on performance items. The purpose of these explorations is to determine the student's level of performance under more nearly optimal conditions, or to reduce the effects of conditions that are hypothesized to obstruct performance. When a dynamic assessment is carried out, there is no other agenda for that session other than to work on that approach; it is not "tacked onto" another approach. The assessor enters the session with the idea that the next one to several hours will be totally dedicated to exploring the learner's responsivity in a considerably more intensive and systematic way than would be possible by means of testing limits.

Dynamic assessment contrasts with diagnostic teaching in its focus on cognitive functions and processes (e.g., attention maintenance, impulse regulation, strategy application) rather than on curriculum content. Of course, any process is embedded in content, and any process is best explored in terms of consistency or inconsistency across content. However, dynamic assessors are interested in the metacognitive processes of problem solving, as well as in the extent to which the learner's metacognitive abilities can be enhanced.

EARLY HISTORY

Despite the fact that dynamic assessment is a relatively new addition to the diagnostic repertory, it has a history that dates back at least to the beginning of the 20th century. The theoretical roots for dynamic assessment can be traced to Vygotsky's conceptualization of the "zone of proximal development" (ZPD; see Minick, 1987, for a thorough discussion). The ZPD concept refers to the idea that a child has some fully matured processes that are evident when the child is assessed by traditional means, as well as emergent developmental processes that can become evident when the child interacts with a more knowledgeable partner. The ZPD is the difference between the child's level of performance when functioning independently and the child's level of performance when functioning in collaboration with a more knowledgeable partner. This can also be viewed as a definition of "potential." Although Vygotsky did not live long enough to realize ZPD in an assessment procedure, the concept of ZPD remains a very powerful stimulus for those who are interested in developing these approaches.

The ongoing challenge is to determine means of interacting in a facilitative manner with the child so as to maximize the ZPD, or at least to devise means of effectively revealing these capacities. This is discussed at greater length in Part II of this book.

Aside from Vygotsky, the historical foundations of dynamic assessment have been mostly pragmatic. Since the writings of Dearborn (1921) and Penrose (1934), there have been complaints regarding definitions of intelligence that omit inclusion of the ability to learn, and proposals that measures of this ability would more accurately reflect intelligence. Elsewhere (Lidz, 1987b), I have provided a detailed accounting of the history of dynamic assessment. However, three consistent findings are particularly worthy of mention. First is the idea that practice alone has not been successful in producing improvement in cognitive functioning, in contrast to the considerably greater support for the positive effects of intervention strategies that include elaboration and mediation (these concepts are discussed in greater detail later). Second is the finding of the greater predictive power of "posttraining" scores — that is, of learner performance following provision of intervention. Third is the evidence for the enhanced modifiability of subjects with low initial levels of performance under "enriched" conditions of presenting material. Special mention should be made of Binet and Simon (1916/1980), who, despite having "fathered" the traditional IQ test, did not adhere to a concept of fixed intelligence.

Studies by researchers such as Rohwer and Ammon (1971) and Carlson and Wiedl (1980) have provided impressive evidence of the superiority of elaborated feedback and mediational interventions over practice and familiarization alone for increasing learners' performance on tests, particularly for subjects with relatively low levels of initial performance. Such feedback not only provides information to the learner about the correctness of performance, but includes a general rule or principle underlying successful performance. DeWeerdt (1927), Schucman (1960), and Bailey (1981) offer evidence of improved predictive power of posttraining as compared with pretraining test scores (in Bailey's study, this difference did not reach statistical significance, but the trend was evident for 13 of their 16 subjects). Finally, studies by Gordon and Haywood (1969) and Haywood and Switzky (1974) are examples of the improved ability of low-functioning subjects to respond at previously unanticipated levels when offered enriched presentations of materials — in these cases, of an increased number of exemplars for a reasoning task involving determination of similarities among a number of items within a category.

Historical pioneers of dynamic-like assessment procedures include Ortar (1959) in Israel, and both Haeussermann (1958) and Schucman

(1960) in the United States. Ortar was interested in determining educability. Both Haeussermann and Schucman designed their procedures for the assessment of severely dysfunctional children (in Schucman's case, mentally deficient; in Haeussermann's, cerebral-palsied). Haeussermann provided a number of probes to determine at what level and by what means a child not otherwise able to succeed could be helped to respond successfully; she devised her complex and nonstandardized approach for use with children during their preschool years. Schucman was particularly interested in a child's ability to transfer and retain learning, and provided retests after periods of 1 hour, 1 week, and 7 weeks. Working with children between the ages of 5 years, 1 month and 11 years, 1 month, she designed a battery of five nonverbal tests that tapped imitative ability, memory, and discrimination of size, brightness, and shapes.

Although dynamic assessment is clearly a model with implied procedures, this approach to assessment goes beyond mere procedures, and represents an attitude as well. Dynamic assessors are convinced that children can learn if sufficient time and effort is expended to discover the means by which they can profit from intervention. Dynamic assessors are also more interested in spending this time to derive ideas for intervention rather than for placement or classification decisions. The focus of dynamic assessment is on the assessor's ability to discover the means of facilitating the learning of the child, not on the child's demonstration of ability to the assessor. Although assessment of process has acquired a bad reputation over the last several years, there is increasing evidence of the importance of metacognitive processes and the validity of teaching strategies (to be discussed in a later chapter). Designers of dynamic assessment procedures do attempt to address the processes that appear to underlie successful task performance within and across a variety of content domains.

2

Prevailing Dynamic Assessment Models: Feuerstein's Learning Potential Assessment Device

Three prevailing models dominate the dynamic assessment literature in English: Feuerstein's, Brown and Campione's, and Budoff's. Although all share some common features — primarily their interest in assessing learner modifiability by means of a test–intervene–retest format — there are considerable differences. The next two chapters review these models, and offer a critique and discussion regarding applicability of each. Research on each model is discussed in Chapter 5; however, the research relating to psychometric properties of the instruments involved is described in the chapters in which they are introduced. Feuerstein's model is discussed here; the other two are covered in Chapter 3.

Reuven Feuerstein's work with low-performing children dates back at least to the early 1950s, following work with André Rey and Jean Piaget at the University of Geneva. Working with adolescents in Israel's Youth Aliyah, he and his colleagues Ya'acov Rand and Mildred Hoffman not only became dissatisfied with the nature of the information yielded by traditional measures, but devised their own, the Learning Potential Assessment Device (LPAD; Feuerstein, 1979). This assessment was soon followed by an intervention, derived from the same theoretical premises: Instrumental Enrichment (Feuerstein, 1980). Based on a theory of "structural cognitive modifiability," the LPAD involves three core concepts. First, the *learner's* behavior is represented in terms of a variety of cognitive deficiencies, found through clinical experience to typify the performance of children with low academic achievement. Second, the *assessor's* behavior is characterized in terms of the components of the Mediated Learning Experience (MLE), hypothesized to represent the proximal (in contrast to distal) factors relating to development of cognitive functions. Third, the *task* is conceptualized in terms of a "cognitive map" that portrays the features distinguishing one task from another. Each of these central ideas is now explained.

THE LEARNER

Feuerstein describes successful versus unsuccessful approaches to learning in terms of a number of cognitive functions and deficiencies that are organized according to an input–elaboration–output model of the mental act. As he is most concerned with improving the performance of unsuccessful performers, these functions are expressed primarily as cognitive deficiencies. The source of these deficiencies is thought to be inadequacies of MLEs, a concept that is elaborated upon below. In any description of the learner during the course of the assessment process, it is the list of cognitive deficiencies that is most relevant, and it is remediation of these deficiencies that is directly addressed by the assessment. Elaborations on the deficiencies are not offered here, as this is not the forum for a full consideration of these models. Readers who are interested in a more detailed description are referred to the primary texts (Feuerstein, 1979, 1980).

Deficiencies at the input phase include processes pertaining to the initial data gathering of the problem-solving process. Deficiencies at the elaboration phase pertain to the individual's ability to use the data gathered during the course of the problem-solving process. Deficiencies at the output phase involve the learner's ability to communicate solutions and responses to the problem-solving process (Feuerstein, Haywood, Rand, Hoffman, & Jensen, no date). Although the names of these deficiencies may sound somewhat esoteric, many are recognizable as characteristics of the learning process discussed in the cognitive literature. Elsewhere (Lidz, 1987b, p. 464) I have summarized the characteristics of a good learner, as derived from a literature review, as follows: A good learner

1. has an adequate knowledge and skill base relevant to the task;
2. spontaneously selects and applies the strategies and processes relevant to the task, adequately monitoring and evaluating the results of efforts;
3. has good memory storage and retrieval;
4. applies strategies and processes in a flexible way;

   5. inhibits impulsivity to allow for adequate comprehension, pro-
      cessing, and development of hypotheses;
   6. functions in an efficient manner, involving automatization of
      subskills and fast speed of processing;
   7. employs a reflective, field-independent, analytical cognitive
      style;
   8. proceeds with a systematic, strategic approach, when appropri-
      ate;
   9. shows active involvement in learning; and
  10. shows concern with adequacy of solutions.

Though stated more positively, and as functions rather than as
deficiencies, these qualities overlap many of the deficiencies described
by Feuerstein et al. (no date) and suggest that there is research support
for much of what is included. In a diagnostic–remedial approach such
as Feuerstein's, there is an inevitable focus on deficient performance,
because these are the types of cases that are referred and brought to the
attention of the assessors. However, it is necessary to have a model of
optimal performance in order to determine what is deficient, and the
combination of the two listings can promote such a reconceptualization,
while joining the research data base with the richness of clinical
observations.

However, some deficiencies included in Feuerstein's system do not
appear in the research literature, but add considerably to our understanding of how poor learners function. "Episodic grasp of reality" is
one example. This term refers to the idea that one aspect of poor
learning is the failure to connect or relate experiences. To many
children (and adults), each event or occurrence of a situation is an event
in and of itself, with no apparent relationship to preceding situations
and without implications for the future; this can also be expressed in
terms of a failure to think in terms of cause and effect. The
consequences of such a deficiency include the inability to analyze
situations so as to understand their origins, with the consequent
inability to develop a feeling of control over one's life and an inability
to plan for the future. This deficiency has direct implications for
intervention, expressed in terms of the component of "bridging" that is
built into intervention programs based on Feuerstein's theories.
Teachers and parents are taught to build in deliberate connections
("bridges") between what is presented or discussed within any single
lesson and other aspects of the student's life, so that the child learns to
see connections between what is happening in the present and what has
happened before, as well as what might be anticipated in the future.
This, then, is an example of the contribution of the more clinical

aspects of this model, as well as of the interrelatedness of the theory with the diagnosis and the intervention.

The objectives of this model of dynamic assessment are to profile the learner's adequacies and deficiencies, to derive an impression of the learner's modifiability, to induce active and self-regulated learning, to determine the level of intensity necessary to produce changes (modifiability and active, self-regulated learning), and to sample interventions that demonstrate effectiveness or lack of effectiveness in inducing improvements in performance.

THE ASSESSOR

The role of the assessor during the course of a dynamic assessment is not only to note the strengths and weaknesses in the child's cognitive processing, but to provide actual interventions related to the content being presented. The assessor strives to function as an optimal teacher, engaging in behaviors that have been found to be definitive of excellence in teaching or parenting (i.e., behaviors that have been associated with optimal cognitive development in children).

The behavior of the assessor during the course of this model of dynamic assessment is describable in terms of the components of the MLE. As mentioned above, MLEs are hypothesized to account for the experiential aspects that influence cognitive development. The concept is offered to explain how some learners develop more adequately than others (given constancies of "nature"). Actually, MLEs are granted even greater power than this. The biological and sociological aspects of the learner are said not to be the direct, or most primary, influence for cognitive development. Biology and sociology function to influence the organism's receptivity to MLEs. Thus, the importance of organismic factors is not denied, and the total onus or "blame" for low cognitive functioning is not placed on the caregiver. Nevertheless, it is the MLE that is viewed as the most proximal factor in this learning model, following direct learning experience.

The learning model is this: Learning takes place in terms of both direct learning experiences and MLEs. Although direct experiences may account for the largest proportion of interactions, MLEs influence the significance and adequacy of these as well. That is, the more nearly optimal the MLEs, the more they enhance the direct experiences. This model modifies Piaget's "stimulus–organism–response" (S-O-R) model by introducing the human/social interaction (H) factor, yielding an S-H-O-H-R model. The social environment filters, focuses, and interprets experiences impinging on the learner, and at a later phase provides the format for response as well.

Given the proposed importance of the MLE, Feuerstein offers a listing of its most potent characteristics. These include the following:

1. *Mediation of intentionality and reciprocity.* The mediator makes a deliberate attempt to influence the performance of the child, and the child shows a willingness to receive this input from the mediator.

2. *Mediation of meaning.* The mediator attributes value and highlights the importance of content through voice modulation and shows of affect; in this way, the task moves from neutral to meaningful in either a positive or negative direction. For example, the mediator helps the task or situation "come alive," and the learner is helped to discriminate between what is and is not important—what to note and what to ignore.

3. *Mediation of transcendence.* The mediator bridges and connects the current, tangible, and perceivable experience to events in the past or future that require visualization and mental operations. For example, the mediator induces abstract "if–then," "what if," or cause-and-effect thinking about the task or experience, moving the learner mentally beyond the concreteness of the immediate experience.

4. *Mediation of feelings of competence.* The mediator manipulates the task or offers encouraging remarks and praise to induce a feeling of competence and mastery within the child. The child is enabled to leave the situation with the conclusion that "I did it; I can succeed."

5. *Mediated regulation and control of behavior.* The mediator helps the child to inhibit impulsive responses, as well as to increase her focus and attention. The optimal state is self-regulation and active, sustained involvement. Thus, the optimal mediation does not stop with inhibition, but goes on to induce self-regulation on the part of the learner.

6. *Mediated sharing behavior.* The mediator communicates a sense of shared experience with the learner, trying to join the learner's perceptions. This can take the form of attempting to see the situation through the eyes of the learner, and of conveying a sense of "we" or "us" in the experience; it may also include an actual sharing of tasks and chores in order to induce cooperation and shared responsibility.

7. *Mediation of individuation and psychological differentiation.* The mediator functions to induce a clear sense of "you versus me" in the experience, with the mediator functioning in the role of facilitator for the child. The poorly differentiated mediator may become overinvolved in the task or experience—at times taking over and forgetting that it is the child's experience, and that the child needs the mediator to maintain the role of resource.

8. *Mediation of goal seeking, setting, planning, and achieving.* The mediator helps the child to become aware of and maintain focus on the

goal or objective of the task, and helps the child to determine effective strategies to reach the goal. This induces projection of thinking into the future and development of strategic thinking, as well as clarity of purpose.

9. *Mediation of challenge.* The mediator helps the child to reach beyond his current level of functioning without becoming overwhelmed. This component can be related to Vygotsky's concept of the "zone of proximal development." The teaching adult helps to create the optimal match between the child's abilities and the situation in which the child is involved; the child initially requires help from the adult, but is helped by the adult to function independently.

10. *Mediation of change.* The adult communicates to the learner that she is indeed a learner, and that there is a difference between the child's level of performance before and after the interaction. The mediator provides the message of modifiability to the child: "You can learn; you can change; you are modifiable in response to your experiences" (and produces the evidence to document this perception).

11. *Mediation of an optimistic alternative.* The mediator conveys the idea to the learner that there is hope; that some choices may lead to positive outcomes; and, most of all, that what the learner does can make a difference to the outcome. This is the antithesis to a fatalistic attitude of passive acceptance.

I have incorporated these components into a rating scale, with some modifications (see Part II of this book). Parts II and III of this book describe the MLE in greater detail, and allow the assessor to use the concept of MLE as a guideline for interactions with the child during the course of the dynamic assessment. The MLE Rating Scale also allows assessment of both parents' and teachers' interactions with children, which can then be related to prescriptions for intervention. The scale can also serve as an assessment of response to intervention, and in this way functions as a curriculum-based procedure.

One behavior that is not "mediational" in nature, but nevertheless is necessary to the assessment interaction, is the teaching of content necessary for the task. The assessor needs to broaden the learner's knowledge base so that he has the tools for dealing with the task. It is the way this is done that may be mediational, although direct instruction and nonmediational practice may be involved as well. Not every aspect of the interaction is mediational; the objective of mediated interventions is to promote independent, representational problem-solving abilities. It should be possible to detect examples of the MLE components when viewing the overall interaction, even if not every element of the interaction falls within the MLE categories.

We now have a way to describe the characteristics of the learner and assessor during the course of the assessment situation. What is needed is a way to characterize the task.

THE TASK

The task within the LPAD model is described here in two ways. First, the actual instruments used in administering the LPAD are briefly discussed; second, the theoretical model used to derive and describe these instruments is outlined. Feuerstein and his colleagues are committed to the idea that the instruments should not duplicate actual achievement tasks within the learner's experience, although the cognitive demands should be generalizable to tasks within similar domains.

The specific instruments that have been incorporated into the LPAD battery include a wide variety of verbal and nonverbal tasks, tapping operations such as analogical reasoning, numerical reasoning, categorization, and memory strategies. Some of these were designed by the LPAD authors; others were adapted from previously designed procedures, many of these by André Rey. A limited selection of these instruments is usually offered. Most are administratable in both an individual and a group format. Instructions are necessarily more standardized and less individually sensitive when the group procedures are administered; however, speed and efficiency are gained. Therefore, the group procedure is used primarily as a screening device to determine students in need of more intensive assessment. The group procedure can also be used to derive educationally prescriptive information that may be more useful than normative results for students with only mild needs, or for guidance of large-group lesson planning. Administration of an LPAD battery, even when administered in the group format, will usually require many hours (easily 5 to 8), although time can be reduced by selecting fewer procedures. However, sufficient time is needed to allow assessment of the learners' modifiability and to facilitate generalization of learning across domains (as well as to gain understanding of pervasiveness of deficiencies across domains). The instruments are described in detail in the manual (Feuerstein et al., no date), and extensive training is required in order to develop proficiency in their administration.

Feuerstein describes his theoretical model of the "cognitive map" to permit analysis and description of the LPAD instruments, and to serve as an outline for designing additional procedures. The cognitive map comprises seven dimensions on which the mental act can be described. Each of these is an area that is manipulable in the assessment or instructional situation. The first dimension is the specific *content* of interest (e.g., math, science, reading, matrices, social comprehension). The second dimension is the *modality* in which the content is presented. This may be verbal, pictorial, numerical, figural, symbolic, graphic, or any combination of these. The third dimension is the *phase of the mental act* (input, elaboration, or output; within a language-based model, these are conceptualizable as reception, processing, or expression). The fourth dimension, the *cognitive operations*, includes such activities as categorization, identification, comparison, seriation, multiplication, permutation, analogical reasoning, and so on; these answer the question of what actually needs to be done in the activity. The fifth dimension is the *level of complexity*, which varies in terms of number of units of information and extent of familiarity with the task demands and content. The sixth dimension, *level of abstraction*, refers to the conceptual distance between the object and the mental operations required, or degree of concreteness. And, finally, the seventh dimension, *level of efficiency*, concerns the issues of speed and accuracy of the mental act: Some activities are best suited for high speed and require a high level of precision, whereas others are best performed slowly and do not necessarily involve high levels of accuracy. This can be illustrated by comparing the skills involved in surgery to those involved in shopping for the week's groceries; determination of competencies in each of these areas would vary considerably on the dimension of level of efficiency.

Analyzing tasks on these dimensions (see Part III of this book, for example) allows comparisons across tasks, and facilitates analysis of an individual's performance on any selection of activities. Using these dimensions enhances the assessor's ability to predict the generalizability of assessment results to the instructional situation. The results should be most generalizable to classroom tasks that share dimensional descriptors. It is also possible for the assessor to administer tasks that overlap with activities in which the student is showing difficulty. In fact, the usefulness of this dimensional outline is not restricted to use with the LPAD, but can be applied outside the dynamic assessment situation as well. (See the curriculum-based adaptation in Part III.)

The major components of the LPAD procedure, involving the learner, the assessor, and the task, have now been described. As can be imagined, putting these pieces together in an actual assessment is a complex process. The LPAD is designed as a clinical procedure, not a standardized or normative one, and, considerable clinical judgment and inference are involved. However, it is not quite so impossible or overwhelming to master as might be suspected upon initial reading. It is particularly important in learning this type of procedure to have access to good models and experienced supervision. Practitioners who wish to become more informed about and to gain experience with this procedure are encouraged first to read the basic books in the area (e.g., Feuerstein, 1979; Lidz, 1987a), and then to attend one of the workshops.

CRITIQUE

The LPAD is the most comprehensive and theoretically grounded expression of the dynamic assessment model to date. It has served as a catalyst for conceptualization and instrument development.

By design, the LPAD is limited to application to older children (aged 9 to 18) and to adults. To say that it is time-consuming is a description and not an evaluation. Despite the behavior and attitudes of some assessors, faster is not necessarily better. Nevertheless, the LPAD, by any standard, is not the procedure of choice for every child who requires diagnostic assessment. The evaluative criteria of usefulness and uniqueness of information yielded, in relation to time required for administration, remain to be determined. The aspect of uniqueness appears most assured, as nondynamic approaches make no claims to information regarding responsiveness to intervention. Although the group administration allows application to larger numbers of children for briefer periods of time, the number of hours required exceed the typical time involvements expected by American consumers.

There are two areas in particular need of further development. One concerns the issue of psychometrics — not necessarily in traditional terms, but psychometrics nevertheless; the second involves the linkage to classroom parameters.

Certain concepts of traditional psychometrics clearly do not apply to dynamic assessment in general and to the LPAD in particular. These include, for example, test–retest reliability and traditional criteria for concurrent and predictive validity. Clearly, a test yielding high stability from time 1 to time 2 is, by definition, not dynamic. The word "dynamic" implies change and not stability. This relates to the choice of items and tests as well. Items on traditional measures are *deliberately* selected to maximize stability, not necessarily to provide an accurate reflection of stability or change in the "real" world. Conversely, procedures selected for dynamic assessment need to be sensitive to change. These two approaches serve very different purposes and reflect very different assumptions and points of view. Similarly, criteria for concurrent and predictive validity need to be relevant for dynamic purposes and concepts, and need therefore to reflect process and not product. Prediction of responsiveness to interventions derived from the assessment is a relevant criterion; static achievement test scores are not.

Nevertheless, reliability and validity are relevant issues for both dynamic and static assessment, and some traditional applications of reliability (such as internal consistency and interrater agreement) have been applied successfully. However, more needs to be done, and more needs to be conceptualized. Some concepts are relevant to static assessment as well. For example, shouldn't all assessment be evaluated in terms of relevance of outcome for the educational setting? And shouldn't all assessment be evaluated in terms of examiners' agreement regarding diagnoses and recommendations? Dynamic assessment needs to proceed in these directions, but then so does static assessment.

The second area related to validity, as mentioned above, is the need to demonstrate linkage to educational variables. The LPAD tests were deliberately selected not to overlap directly with classroom achievement tasks; however, at some point there is a need to provide a more concrete, specific bridge to these tasks, or at least to describe more clearly the procedures for deriving such a bridge. Feuerstein's recent expressions of intent to deal with reading content seem to acknowledge this need. One way to make such a bridge is to have the teacher observe and contribute to the assessment (when she is not the primary assessor), so that linkages can be discussed on a continuing basis during the course of the assessment. This, of course, imposes another time-consuming parameter that many settings may not be able to accommodate. Another possibility is to develop a continuum of tasks that increasingly approximate actual classroom content. Yet another approach is to select actual classroom content relevant to the needs of the referred child, and to incorporate these into a general dynamic assessment model. This is the approach I have chosen, which is described in Part III in application to preschool children.

Finally, some comments apply specifically to the LPAD, particularly to the group procedures. There is some inconsistency regarding the imposition of a test–intervene–retest format. The ability to compare pre- and postintervention performance is an important ingredient of this model, and this aspect of the group administration seems to need some tightening. Also, more information about the psychometric properties of the instruments used for pretesting and posttesting would be helpful. For example, more information is needed regarding what processes are tapped by the tests and to what ages they best apply; most of all, information about the properties of the tests as posttests is needed. Furthermore, definitions of cognitive deficiencies and mediational components would profit from clarification and further definition. Bringing these into line with current research on cognition and educational intervention would also be useful. And finally, training in these procedures needs to be made more widely available and less prohibitively lengthy and expensive. If the procedures are to be used, they need to be taught in the training institutions and expressed in terms of the effective teaching practices that good teachers and parents have been using all along.

3

Prevailing Dynamic Assessment Models, Continued: The Work of Budoff and of Campione and Brown

Feuerstein's LPAD has been presented in Chapter 2 as the most learner-responsive of the prevailing dynamic assessment models, and the most extensive in terms of theoretical elaboration. This chapter describes and discusses two models that share the characteristic of standardization of the intervention phase of the test–intervene–retest model. The designers of these models have chosen the route of increased control and greater ease of generation of psychometric properties. The work of Milton Budoff and his colleagues in Cambridge, Massachusetts, took place between the mid-1960s and the late 1970s. That of Ann L. Brown and Joseph C. Campione and their students and colleagues, first at the University of Illinois and more recently at the University of California–Berkeley, continues to the present. Both groups have made notable contributions to dynamic assessment in their rich and extensive research.

BUDOFF'S LEARNING POTENTIAL ASSESSMENT

Rationale

Quite in contrast to Feuerstein, Budoff and his associates explicitly designed their procedures to serve as an alternative to IQ tests in classifying children for special education purposes. Their concern was to provide a means for more accurate classification of students whose abilities were likely to be underestimated by traditional IQ tests — specifically, minority-group children and those from non-English-dominant homes. Budoff utilizes Raven's Progressive Matrices, as does Feuerstein, as one of his learning potential measures; however, he deviates from Feuerstein in the classification focus, in the standardization of the intervention, and in his less theoretical approach to the assessment. Budoff's intervention more closely approximates a standardized coaching procedure that aims at familiarizing the student with the test demands, thus attempting to equalize the experience of students. Like Feuerstein, and in contrast to Campione and Brown, Budoff chooses to emphasize tasks that are minimally related to academic content, preferring to assess the child's ability to profit from "experience" rather than demonstrate the already apparent school failure. Budoff and his colleagues refer to their approach as "learning potential assessment" (LPA).

Specific Measures

The specific measures of Budoff's LPA have included the Kohs Learning Potential Task (KLPT), the Raven Learning Potential Test (RLPT), the Series Learning Potential Test (SLPT), and the Picture Word Game (PWG). These procedures and related research are described in detail elsewhere (Budoff, 1987a, 1987b). These tests can be administered in both an individual and a group format.

The KLPT is very similar to the Block Design task of the Wechsler tests, although the sides include blue and yellow, as well as red and white, alternatives. The KLPT includes 15 designs, utilizing up to 16 blocks. Budoff has equated the size of the drawings with the blocks by doubling the scale of the drawings on the stimulus cards. The designs used during the training phase consist of three four-block designs from the Wechsler Intelligence Scale for Children (WISC), and two nine-block designs, one from the WISC and one from the Wechsler Adult Intelligence Scale (WAIS). The entire series is administered three times — first, with standard instructions, prior to training; again, with standard instructions, 1 day following training; and sometimes 1 month following training. The training employs progressive simplification: First, the training series is presented without differentiating lines; if these are not solved, the rows of the design are presented one at a time; and if the student still does not succeed, the blocks are all outlined. In addition, praise and encouragement are offered, as well as a model-checking strategy and a concept-building technique for how to build a stripe with two blocks. The KLPT is most appropriately used with students above ages 12 to 13.

The RLPT utilizes the standard administration of Raven's Matrices as a pre- and posttraining measure. The form of the test used varies with the student's age and linguistic background; any of the available formats can be used. The intervening training is recommended to take place over 2 days. The training is carried out on designs that are similar to, but do not duplicate, the actual Raven drawings. During the training, students initially draw the solutions, learning to derive and then draw the specific attribute to be noted. They then move to mental solution of the problems, and learn to verbalize how the solution was derived. The examiner's role is to direct a student's attention; to explain the attributes to be noted; and to guide the student from concrete, motor responses to increasingly abstract conceptualizations. Concepts of perceptual closure, spatial orientation, and double classification are explicitly taught. The student's active involvement is promoted, and praise and encouragement are freely offered. The standardization of the training is approximate and not absolute; the training is estimated to require a total of about 2 hours, comprised of four 30-minute sessions (pretest, two training sessions, and posttest). The RLPT is applicable to children from the ages of 5 through 12 (it can also be used with adolescents), and comes in English and Spanish versions. The stimulus materials are available on slides.

Studies of the RLPT with educable mentally retarded (EMR) and regular education students with ages ranging from 7 through 15 show high internal consistency for both pre- and posttraining tests, as well as low measurement error (Budoff, 1987b). Budoff's research institute has studied 12-year-old students of low socioeconomic status (SES) and has demonstrated that training does improve scores for both special and regular education children. Special education research subjects have not shown transfer beyond the types of problem solution for which they have been trained (Budoff, 1987b).

The 65-item SLPT was designed by Elisha Babad as a group-administered nonverbal reasoning task for students in grades 1 through 3. The test presents a series of pictures that vary four concepts (semantic content, size, color, or spatial orientation); there is a blank space to be filled in from a selection of alternatives, and this blank space may appear anywhere in the series. This test includes an alternate form, used for postintervention testing. Training emphasizes identifying the relevant concepts, detecting the pattern being presented, reversing the pattern when appropriate, and the specific strategy of crossing out alternatives as they are ruled out.

A test–retest reliability study with students from five Connecticut towns (Budoff, 1987b) yielded coefficients of .80 and above for all but one Form B subtest, and for one of the four Form A subtests (Picture Series was the highest in both forms, and Picture Matrix the lowest), with total test score coefficients of .87 and .90 for Forms A and B, respectively. Internal consistency coefficients for both forms were .95. In a factor analysis, only Picture Series emerged as a factor over both forms; however, the factor structures of each form showed differences, with Picture Series accounting for most of the variance in Form A, and a Geometric factor for most of the variance in Form B. Factor analysis of the forms after training yielded structures similar to pretraining Form B. Although students at all grade levels tested (1 through 4) showed improvement with training, the effects of training were most potent for students in grades 1 and 2, and least potent for students in grade 4. The correlation between Forms A and B is reported as .84. IQ was a better predictor than SLPT scores of reading test performance.

The SLPT is concluded to be more sensitive to race and SES than the other measures used by Budoff and his associates; therefore, they conclude, it is a less successful indicator of learning potential. The test appears most useful when used to assess learning potential for low-SES students in grades 2 and 3, and to demonstrate the effects of training for middle-class students in grades 1 and 2. Despite the limitations, Budoff reports that the posttraining scores of his low-SES subjects reached the level of the pretraining scores of his middle-class subjects in four out of five of the Connecticut towns studied.

The PWG, adapted from Rulon's Semantic Test of Intelligence, is appropriate for use with students in kindergarten through grade 2, and involves learning to associate a symbol with a concept derivable from a series of pictures (or a picture with a concept derivable from a series of symbols); in other words, it is a verbal reasoning ability task. For example, a square represents the concept "boy," since all four pictures portray a boy in varying postures. The student must determine, from analysis of the four subsequent pictures, what the stimulus symbol stands for. The PWG does not incorporate a pretest, but moves from training to testing.

The PWG involves 37 items, with half requiring translation from picture to symbol, and half from symbol to picture. It can be administered within one classroom period and to class-size groups. The training episode uses slides and teaches the prerequisite problem-solving strategy, as well as providing familiarity with the task components and experiences of successful problem solution. A study of an early version with 205 low-income urban Massachusetts students (Budoff, 1987b) produced an internal consistency coefficient of .95, with a ceiling effect at or beyond grade 3. A study of the final version

with 90 low-income Massachusetts students (Budoff, 1987b) demonstrated high indices of discrimination for most items, with internal
consistency of .93, and a ceiling effect beyond grade 3. Validity as a
verbal measure was assessed by correlation with the Comprehension
and Vocabulary subtests of the Stanford Achievement Test, yielding
coefficients of .37 and .34, respectively.

Table 3.1 summarizes the age ranges for which each of Budoff's
procedures is most appropriate. As indicated in the table, most of the
procedures are appropriate for children of elementary school age, with
all but the KLPT applicable to young children in the lower primary
grades.

Budoff also presents data to show the following:

1. Higher correlations of KLPT pretraining than posttraining scores
   with IQ for retarded subjects (Hamilton & Budoff, 1974; Budoff
   & Hamilton, 1976).
2. High agreement (16 of 20) of learning potential category with
   teacher indications of learning rate for retarded subjects (Hamilton & Budoff, 1974; Budoff & Hamilton, 1976).
3. Better response of high- than low-SES subjects to the group (as
   opposed to the individual) format (Budoff & Corman, 1973).
4. The most potent aspect of training: provision of a verbal explanation of the problem's critical features (Budoff & Allen, 1978).

Determination of appropriate criteria for predictive validity studies
presents a particular challenge for researchers of dynamic assessment.
Budoff's group has produced two of the few studies that have used a
process, rather than a static, predictive criterion. In a study by Budoff,
Meskin, and Harrison (1971) using an electricity curriculum unit, the
students (some of whom were in regular and some in special education)
were differentiable by classroom assignment on the curriculum pretest.
However, these students could not be differentiated by classroom
assignment following instruction; their posttest scores related only to

TABLE 3.1. Age Ranges for Budoff's LPA Procedures

Procedure	Age range
KLPT	12 to 13 years
RLPT	5 to 12 years
SLPT	6 to 8 years
PWG	5 to 7 years

their learning potential status. Budoff, Corman, and Gimon (1976) assessed 54 Spanish-speaking 6- to 13-year-old students involved in the electricity curriculum unit. Their precurriculum cognitive level was tested in Spanish on the WISC, the Semantic Test of Intelligence, and the RLPT. Only the posttraining scores on the RLPT significantly predicted the postteaching curriculum-based scores.

Critique

Budoff and associates' early work with LPA yielded classification categories of "high scorer" (initially high performance), "gainer" (improvement beyond a preset criterion level in response to training), and "nongainer" (no improvement or below-criterion-level gain following training). However, the researchers could not resolve the issue of the lack of a common point of reference, or that of the determination of the meaning of "gain" vis-à-vis "level of performance." That is, how can performances of two individuals be compared if one starts at a higher point and makes little gain, and the other starts at a lower level, makes a large gain, and either does or does not reach the level of performance of the first child?

This raises an issue that needs to be addressed by all who deal with dynamic assessment: the issue of trying to understand or put into context just what "responsiveness" or "learning" is. It is not unusual to find children at average or better levels of performance on cognitive measures who are not quickly responsive to attempts at short-term intervention, while, conversely, others at comparatively lower levels (even "retarded" levels) of performance demonstrate high degrees of response. It is likely that we are dealing with a dimension, a "trait," or a behavior that may relate to, but may not totally coincide with, cognitive level as indicated by IQ. However, this dimension may be no less an aspect of intelligence, particularly in relation to an instructional environment. Our definitions and comprehension of intelligence may well be enhanced by the addition of "learning ability," rather than by attempts to demonstrate the validity of learning ability in terms of static notions of IQ. This suggests that intelligence is more than what is measured by intelligence tests, or, rather, that intelligence tests may need to measure more.

What is evident is that neither so-called "retarded" nor "nonretarded" groups of children are homogeneous in terms of response to instruction, and there is overlap even in levels of performance, depending upon the nature of the task's demands. The issue does remain, however, that although dropping the "gainer" and "nongainer" categories solves the research problems, the ability to interpret the meaning of score improvements for an individual child is not thereby increased. What becomes necessary is to develop norms for a variety of subgroups so that the meaning of score changes can be enhanced. The result would then be a new type of normed psychometric measure. What is missing is evidence that Budoff's LPA procedures contribute more to predictions of school success than do measures of nonverbal IQ. This is especially important in view of the emphasis of this approach on classification, and the increased time required to administer the procedures.

Despite Budoff's attempts to approach standardization of the training segment, and his criticism of Feuerstein for lack of such standardization (personal communication, 1986) when discussing the need to link assessment with intervention, his approach closely resembles that of Feuerstein:

> In formulating an assessment strategy, the client's strengths and weaknesses should be ascertained in the initial testing contacts or from the referral. . . . Appropriate training and posttest(s) to test hypotheses would then be designed/selected. Subsequent contacts would be used to test and generate hypotheses, and, finally, formulate a treatment plan. (1987a, p. 78)

Specific links to intervention have not been worked out, however, and it remains for others to do this. Furthermore, the lack of explicit links to a theoretical base makes it difficult to analyze the student's performance and the assessor's interventions, in order to facilitate the relationship between assessment and intervention. Budoff's approaches also appear to emphasize the disclosure of already existing abilities, providing an opportunity to equalize experiences related to the tasks, as well as to increase motivation level in relation to task solution. This differs from Feuerstein's attempts to change the child's cognitive functions and to assess the child's responsiveness to attempts at a profound enhancement of problem-solving abilities. Whether such an objective is either meaningful or realistic remains moot. Also, the focus of the Budoff-based assessment is on test analysis rather than on child analysis. Assessors trained in traditional approaches will no doubt feel more comfortable with Budoff's than with Feuerstein's approach, because less demand is placed on the specialist's ability to analyze the ongoing interaction and to modify task administration in response to this analysis; task administration is more controlled and standardized. For these same reasons, Budoff's approach has been more readily incorporated into research studies.

CAMPIONE AND BROWN'S APPROACH

Rationale and Description

Campione and Brown, formerly at the University of Illinois and recently relocated to the University of California–Berkeley, are active and prolific researchers in the area of dynamic assessment. Like others who have been motivated to seek alternatives to traditional cognitive assessment procedures, they are dissatisfied with the limited information provided by normative approaches. They also offer criticism of these traditional measures as underestimating children who have not had preparatory opportunities. Their direction was initially based on their interpretation of the theories and practices of Soviet psychologists such as Vygotsky, particularly regarding the posited importance of socially mediated learning and conceptualization of a "zone of proximal development." They have also been influenced by the literature on instruction and the development of expertise, as well as their own studies regarding metacognition. Campione and Brown share Budoff's objective of standardization and quantification of dynamic assessment, and the focus on analysis of the task rather than the learner. With Feuerstein, they share a focus on process. Their most recent involvement with reciprocal teaching more closely resembles Feuerstein's clinical methods than does their earlier work.

Their most significant contribution has been to attempt a direct linkage between dynamic assessment of processes and achievement content; they strongly advocate the need to embed their approach to assessment in academic content. The processes emphasized are learning and transfer, each operationalized in terms of the number of hints or prompts needed to achieve a criterion (e.g., two items) of independent performance. Information yielded from this approach describes the child's efficiency of learning in terms of number of prompts, and breadth of transfer in terms of degree of success with maintenance, near-transfer, and far-transfer problems. This information describes the amount of help needed by the child, rather than the amount of improvement made by the child in response to the help provided. Budoff's approach provides standardized help and looks at the child's gains. Feuerstein provides unstandardized help and also looks at the child's response, further analyzing the types of help provided and the complexities of the child's responses.

The specific tasks used in the research of Campione and Brown and their students (e.g., Bryant, 1982; Campione, Brown, & Bryant, 1985; Campione, Brown, Ferrara, Jones, & Steinberg, 1985) include matrices and letter completion (in their earlier studies), and beginning levels of reading and math (in their later studies). The typical sequence includes three to four sessions, with the following activities: collection of static, level-of-performance information; initial mediated learning; static, unmediated maintenance and transfer assessment; mediated maintenance and transfer assessment. Mediation in this context includes provision of predetermined hints, in a graduated sequence from the most general to the most specific (and, finally, to task completion by the examiner). A new hint is provided in response to indications of struggle, failure, or error on the part of the child; provision of hints is terminated when the child achieves the level of independent task solution preset for the task, such as two consecutive items. Mediated maintenance and transfer sessions also include provision of the same gradient of hints. The metric yielded from this procedure is a sum of the total number of hints provided for each segment (e.g., initial learning, maintenance, transfer) of the task.

Campione and Brown's dynamic-assessment-related research began by addressing psychometric issues — specifically, with an investigation of concurrent and predictive validity. Evidence for concurrent validity was provided by the findings that younger and lower-IQ children performed more poorly on the dynamic assessment procedures, and that both maintenance and transfer scores accurately differentiated retarded from nonretarded performers. Support for predictive validity was derived from the outprediction of gain scores on academic tests of static scores by both learning and transfer scores, with far transfer being the most powerful contributor to prediction of performance. Learning and transfer scores added from 22% to 40% variance to static scores. Their research also documented significant moderate-level correlations of learning performance across tasks, with a tendency toward higher learning consistency than transfer consistency. On the basis of these results, Campione and Brown (1990) conclude: "If the interest is in predicting the learning trajectory of different students, the best indicant is not their IQ or how much they know originally, nor even how readily they acquire new procedures, but how well they understand and make flexible use of those procedures in the service of solving novel problems" (pp. 164–165).

Critique

The Campione and Brown approach to dynamic assessment, because of its relative ease of quantification, has generated a number of interesting and important research studies. These researchers not only have documented the contributions of a dynamic, process-oriented approach to prediction of children's cognitive performance, but have also been successful in embedding the procedures in early mastery aspects of academic content.

Several questions and issues apply to these procedures. Of greatest concern is the nature and meaning of the metric generated by the prompting procedures—essentially, a sum total of the number of prompts required to reach independent problem solution. Such an approach suggests that the prompt gradient forms a scale, and includes inferences that the hierarchy reflects level of complexity, that each step is relatively equal, and that it is the quantity rather than the nature of the intervention that is relevant to learning. These inferences remain to be investigated. The guiding principle for inclusion of a prompt appears to be the degree of generality versus specificity, rather than the nature of metacognitive processes to be facilitated or addressed; a theory of learning or instruction is not apparent in the derivation or application of the prompts. Furthermore, there appears to be no calculation of changes in need for prompts across items within a problem type—information that could be available from this approach, and perhaps even more relevant to estimations of acquisition and transfer than the current metric. The focus on the task rather than the learner's responsiveness limits the diagnostic usefulness of this approach, although the research using this approach may be quite relevant for instructional practices and for programming computer tutorials for children with mild mastery deficits.

The qualitative nature of the Campione and Brown prompting intervention is quite different from the mediation provided in Feuerstein's approach, although both are referred to as "mediation," and both have roots in Vygotsky's work. The Campione and Brown mediation appears to emphasize the focusing of attention on cues and patterns relevant for problem solution; the assessor works up to total demonstration, but not necessarily to explanation. Their later work includes memory jogs and suggestions of the need to strategize. Feuerstein's conceptualization of mediation is considerably more comprehensive and complex (see Part II of this book). For example, it involves components of meaning and transcendence that find support in the instructional research literature. The students are given more than reminders; they are provided with expanded explanations and principles of problem solution. There is no inherent reason why such components could not be included in the prompting hierarchy; they are merely not apparent at this time. Further study regarding the types of prompts that are most effective and for whom is warranted (research of this type has been carried out by Carlson & Wiedl, 1980). Such modifications would provide much-needed diagnostic information. In its current form, the procedure is more relevant for input into decisions relating to classification and determination of academic mastery than for input into decisions regarding interventions.

Children who do not achieve a criterion level of independent functioning are disqualified from inclusion in the studies by Campione and Brown and their colleagues. The possible effects of this on their research results warrant further analysis and discussion. For example, such exclusions would seem to restrict the applicability of the procedure to certain levels of performance.

There is also an issue regarding the types of tasks to which the Campione and Brown approach is relevant. Thus far, the nature of the tasks has been low-level, initial mastery when the content domain has been academic. Interestingly, when more complex content (reading comprehension) has been involved, the procedure applied has become more clinical (i.e., reciprocal teaching; Palincsar & Brown, 1984).

The Campione and Brown research has been very central in highlighting the importance of including near-transfer, and particularly far-transfer, information in assessment; this inclusion is relevant for static as well as dynamic assessments. An optimal assessment approach that focuses on abilities of individuals, based on the approaches designed by the three major groups of contributors to dynamic assessment procedure design, would include the following components: establishment of level of performance, determination of modifiability and response to instruction within the same domain, diagnostic clues regarding potentially effective instructional strategies, and indications of ability to maintain and transfer what was learned. In this way, when the questions posed are "What does this child know now; what are his learning gaps (process and content); and how can he best be taught?", the assessment responses are provided from the combined application of normed, curriculum-referenced, and dynamic strategies.

4

Dynamic Assessment Applied to Preschool Children

Dynamic assessment procedures were initially developed for use with school-age children and adolescents. Feuerstein's LPAD has been applied with children as young as 9 to 10 years, and Mearig (1987) has designed a downward extension of the LPAD for use with children from the ages of 5 through 8. Budoff's procedures have been used with children as young as age 5, and the students of Campione and Brown have applied their approach with children as young as age 4. However, none of these approaches is considered explicitly a "preschool" procedure.

This chapter focuses on procedures and related research that have been developed specifically for use with very young children — that is, children between the ages of 4 through 6 years. I have been one of the contributors to the endeavor of designing a downward extension of the dynamic assessment model to very young children, and this approach is described in detail in Part III of this book; therefore, it is not elaborated upon here.

One of the defining characteristics of dynamic assessment is the focus on cognitive processes rather than products related to learning — specifically, on metacognitive processes. Such a focus raises the question of the appropriateness of these procedures with young children. Most developmentalists would likely agree that children are not born with fully developed metacognition, and that although a "dynamic-like" diagnostic approach may be possible at any age, a true "dynamic" assessment seems applicable only to children with at least emerging metacognitive processing capabilities. In a review of the cognitive functioning of preschool children, we (Lidz & Thomas, 1987) concluded that although the ages of 5 to 6 appears to be of particular significance to the development of metacognitive processing in the normal child, many processes are emerging from the ages of 3 through 5. Such emerging processes include self-regulation, early logic (e.g., identities and functions that permit comparative behavior, prediction of consequences, and means–ends analysis), early deductive reasoning (a shift from visual–motor to visual–figurative to verbal thinking), and some signs of the ability to derive and apply strategies (e.g., regarding perception and memory).

Also, Ballester (1984) demonstrated that some of the cognitive functions (as deficiencies) discussed by Feuerstein could be observed in the performances of preschool children, and that associations could be found between these functions and the children's preschool academic achievement. Spontaneous comparative behavior was the most strongly associated of the functions with achievement for these 4-year-old, low-SES, African-American, urban children.

In addition to myself and my colleagues, the primary procedure designers and researchers in the area of preschool dynamic assessment have been David Tzuriel and Pnina S. Klein of Bar Ilan University in Israel, and M. Susan Burns and her colleagues, first at Vanderbilt University and now at Tulane University.

THE WORK OF TZURIEL AND KLEIN

Tzuriel has codesigned two preschool dynamic assessment procedures with Klein, and is the sole author of a third. The coauthored procedures are the Children's Analogical Thinking Modifiability Test (CATM; Tzuriel & Klein, 1985, 1987) and the Frame Test of Cognitive Modifiability (FTCM; Tzuriel & Klein, 1986). The single-authored procedure is the Children's Inferential Thinking Modifiability Test (CITM; Tzuriel, 1989). These tests all follow a test–intervene–retest format, preceded by a familiarization stage that reviews the dimensions of the materials (e.g., size, color, shape, picture names) and the rules of problem solution (what is required on the task). The pre- and postintervention tests are alternative forms, and the procedures differ in the cognitive functions and operations tapped.

The CATM includes 18 blocks, varying on dimensions of size (large, small), color (red, yellow, blue), and shape (circle, square, triangle). The child is presented with a series of analogical problems of increasing difficulty. A sample problem is as follows: "Small blue square [is to] small blue circle [as] large yellow square [is to] ___?___ ." The intervention or mediation phase, when used for research, is standardized in its coverage of the needs to search for relevant dimensions, to understand transformational and analogical principles, to search systematically for the missing block, and to improve the efficiency of performance. When the CATM is used diagnostically, the examiner is free to provide whatever mediation is judged to be appropriate for the child.

The first reported research using the CATM (Tzuriel & Klein, 1985) included Israeli children between the ages of 4 and $6\frac{1}{2}$ years. Internal consistencies of the pretest and posttest, as determined by Cronbach's alpha, were .72 for the former and .90 for the latter (reliability thus increased following exposure to the mediation phase). Evidence for validity was provided by differential correlations between gain scores for regular, disadvantaged, special education (mixed problems, unclassified, located in regular schools), and mentally retarded (institutionalized) children, in descending order of performance; that is, the regular and disadvantaged children made the most gain, and the special education and mentally retarded children made the least. The low-SES children made the most gain from pretest to posttest. However, when a partial (rather than all-or-none) scoring was used, the mentally retarded children showed gains equal to those of both regular and low-SES children, despite their lower-level performance; in addition, when the partial scoring method was used, the low-SES group scored the highest of any group on total performance, and the performance of the special education students decreased from pretest to posttest. With the exception of the special education students, the performance of all groups improved from pretest to posttest when either scoring method was used.

In a study using the CATM with Canadian special needs preschool children (mean age = 4 years, 8 months), Missiuna (1986) compared the effects on posttesting of a mediational and a standardized intervention phase. The mediational approach provided interventions that were more contingent on a child's perceived responses and difficulties. The standardized intervention followed a predetermined script that included discussion of the method for problem solution, analysis of relevant dimensions, and provision of positive feedback regarding correct solutions. On both the all-or-none and the partial scoring method, the mediated group showed significant improvement, whereas the performance of the standardized teaching group remained unchanged. No additional time was required to provide mediation, but the mediated children took more time during the posttest phase, suggesting that the mediation increased their ability to inhibit impulsivity and promoted reflective thinking.

The FTCM is made up of five $7\frac{1}{2}$-inch square wooden frames and 32 beads, colored red, yellow, blue, and green. The problems presented tap inductive reasoning, and the prerequisite knowledge base includes colors, numbers, and location. The "problem" is set forth in the first three of four frame sequences, with the child providing the "solution" in the fourth. The fifth frame is used only for demonstration purposes during the intervention phase. Problems are presented that involve simultaneous consideration of several elements. For example, a series may begin with one red bead in the upper right corner of frame 1, two red beads in the lower right corner of frame 2, and three red beads in the lower left corner of frame 3. The child must deduce the rule and place four red beads in the upper left corner of frame 4. In this case, it is only number and location that vary, while color is constant. During the intervention phase, the examiner helps the child focus on the relevant elements, deduce the rule, and restrain impulsivity. During this phase, the fifth frame is used to incorporate the entire sequence of moves within one frame to highlight the rule.

Research on the FTCM was carried out by Tzuriel and Klein (no date), using 82 kindergarten children aged 4 and 5, and 20 first-grade children; both groups were from middle-class families. The children were also administered Raven's Coloured Progressive Matrices. The study showed that the FTCM scores increased with age, with post-teaching scores higher than preteaching scores, and with scores on the dimensions of color and number higher than those on location. The intervention was more successful in increasing the location scores than the scores on the other two dimensions. Age differences were greater on the Raven than on the FTCM.

The CITM is Tzuriel's most recent development, and is based on the LPAD test called the Organizer. This procedure taps inferential reasoning. The familiarization stage assesses the child's ability to recognize and name the pictures to be used in the problems. The problems presented involve a series of picture "sentences," each providing partial information about which of the involved pictures belongs in which order in each of several houses. After "reading" the sentences, the child is asked to infer to which houses the pictures belong. The solution requires combining bits of information accumulated across the sentences; the child learns to develop a hypothesis with one sentence and to confirm it with the succeeding sentences.

Research on the CITM with Israeli kindergarten and first-grade children, including groups of low-SES and middle-class children, is reported in Tzuriel (1989). The low-SES subjects scored significantly lower than the middle-class subjects, and the kindergarten children obtained significantly lower scores than those in first grade. SES was a more potent contributor to the scores of the first-graders. Postteaching scores were significantly higher than preteaching scores for all groups. The kindergarten group showed more improvement than the first-grade group, and the disadvantaged group made more improvement than the middle-class children. In fact, the low-SES children moved from lower-level preteaching scores to a level of postteaching scores similar to that of the middle class; this effect was primarily attributable to the tremendous improvement of the low-SES kindergarten group.

This study also showed significant positive correlations between scores on Raven's Coloured Progressive Matrices (administered as a static test) and both pre- and postteaching scores of the middle-class group, but no relationship between the Raven scores and either the pre- or postteaching CITM scores for the low-SES group. This study also demonstrated that the mediation affected solution of the more complex items, and that the preteaching score was significantly correlated with the postteaching score only in the middle-class group. These findings are similar to those found in the CATM study, and support cross-domain consistency. There appeared to be a ceiling effect only for the first-grade, middle-class group, and only on the posttest; this may have reduced the amount of gain possible for this group, but it would be an unlikely influence on their pattern of performance, since this group began at a higher level and maintained this superiority throughout.

THE WORK OF BURNS AND COLLEAGUES

Burns (1980) has designed two brief (30-minute) procedures that simplify the original Grace Arthur Stencil Design Test (Arthur, 1945) for application to children 4 to 5 years of age. She has also derived a list of behavioral observation categories that have been useful descriptors of young children's problem-solving approaches (Burns, Haywood, Delclos, & Siewert, 1985).

Burns's original Stencil Design Test (SDT) added seven designs to those of the original test, which required only two stencils. There are thus a total of nine designs in the SDT, requiring a total of 18 cards (6 of which are solid colors, and the remaining 12 of which have an area cut out to form a geometric figure). The designs can all be made with two cards, one solid and one cut out. One item is used for demonstration, four for training, and four for pre- and posttesting.

Burns and colleagues (Burns, Vye, Bransford, Delclos, & Ogan, 1987) also designed an Animal Stencil Test of 18 cards, which consists of 6 solid colors (the same as the original SDT) and 12 cut out to form animal shapes. This has been used in research as a near-transfer measure. The mediation provided during the intervention phase of both SDT and Animal Stencil Test administration, when administered dynamically, includes familiarizing the child with the materials and relevant dimensions, teaching the child the rule for combining the stencils (including use of the model), and providing elaborated feedback that includes information regarding what was correct or incorrect about the child's performance (Symons & Vye, 1986).

The first study using the SDT did not involve dynamic administration of the test. This study compared the cognitive approaches of low- and high-SES 4- and 5-year-old children. Effects of gender and race were ruled out. The children were videotaped and their behaviors scored while working on a series of six tasks, one of which was the SDT; it was for this study that the SDT was designed. The frequency of occurrence of 11 child behaviors was determined. These are listed and defined in Vye, Burns, Delclos, and Bransford (1987, p. 343) as follows (10 of the 11 are given here, as number 11 does not apply to the SDT):

1. Attention: looks at examiner or materials during instructions and/or looks at materials while performing.
2. Attention and on-task manipulation: active contact, using hands, with the materials that the child is working on.
3. Off-task behavior: active contact, using hands, on the environment or body that is not part of the material in the study.
4. Information giving: explains what he or she is going to do before performing the task and/or explains intermediate steps.
5. Visual scan/looking at model: looks at model or head moves past the (imaginary) center line dividing the left and right sides of the materials.
6. Corrects self: gives an answer and, without intervention, changes the answer.
7. Confirmation seeking, helpless gestures, and verbalizations: looks to the examiner while using the task materials or asks for help in a nonspecific request.
8. On-task comments: comments made by the child about the task that are not specific to task completion.
9. Inappropriate manipulation of stencils: the number of stencils that the child touches that are not a part of the model design.
10. Speaking out before instructions are finished: speaks, gestures, or starts the task before the instructions are completed.

Although the sources for each of these behaviors are not clearly specified, many relate directly to Feuerstein's list of cognitive deficiencies, and others to the literature on self-regulation. Frequency and duration in seconds were recorded for each behavior, with a median interscorer reliability established at .93, ranging from .79 to .98 (Burns, 1980). There were only three significant differences related to SES on these behaviors: Low-SES children did more confirmation seeking and correcting self, whereas high-SES children did more visual scanning/looking at model. This last finding is similar to the results of the Ballester (1984) study, in which spontaneous comparative behavior (defined as looking at the model) was the most potent aspect of the children's behavior relating to preschool achievement.

In a second study using the SDT, Burns (1985) designed a dynamic assessment format, and compared graduated-prompt and mediational interventions to each other and to static assessment. Each of these was compared in relation to a criterion of postintervention independent performance on the SDT, as well as in relation to a transfer task (Wechsler Preschool and Primary Scale of Intelligence [WPPSI] Animal House). This study involved 60 children between the ages of 4 and 6, with McCarthy Scales General Cognitive Index (GCI) scores between 60 and 89. The children were first pretested on the Animal House; then administered the intervention or given the static SDT, according to their group assignment; then retested for independent performance on the SDT; and then retested on the Animal House. These children were also rated on the behavioral observation scale designed for the earlier study. In relation to the criterion of independent performance on the SDT, there were significant differences between all groups, which performed in the following order: mediated assessment, highest and higher than graduated-prompt assessment; graduated-prompt next and higher than static assessment. In relation to the transfer task, both the mediation and graduated-prompt groups scored higher than the static group, but they did not significantly differ from each other; however, more children in the mediation group reached a criterion level of performance (three out of four correct). There were no significant effects regarding the behavioral observations; however, the observations were scored with .96 interscorer reliability, but with low frequencies of occurrence.

In a study involving preschool children that correlated McCarthy GCI and SDT (graduated-prompt) results, no relationship was found (Vye et al., 1987). Of the McCarthy subscales, only Perceptual–Performance, sharing content domain with the SDT, was related to the results of the dynamic assessment and this correlation was only moderate (.48). The authors interpret this as a failure of static level of performance to predict response to instruction. This is reinforced by their further breakdown of the data to illustrate that substantial numbers of children with GCIs within an "at-risk" range were able to reach a criterion level (three of four correct) of performance on the

SDT (82% with GCIs of 69–108; 53% with GCIs of 53–68; 36% with GCIs of 37–52; and over 25% with GCIs below 37). This is seen as substantiating evidence from other sources that static intelligence indicators provide limited information about children's learning; that children with seemingly similar levels of performance may vary considerably on other learning indicators; and that static and dynamic measures appear to be tapping different characteristics. Vye et al. (1987) also provide evidence of better prediction of within-domain than across-domain transfer. Positive transfer effects were found between the SDT and the Animal Design Test, as well as between the SDT and both a reverse-stencils test and the WPPSI Animal House.

Finally, as a follow-up to their 1985 study, Burns et al. (1987) conducted a second study investigating the differential effects of mediated, graduated-prompt, and static assessment. This study included 44 preschool children with McCarthy GCIs below 70 (mean = 68.75, SD = 10.89). These authors cite a study demonstrating an average performance of one correct on the SDT for children age $5\frac{1}{2}$ years when the SDT is administered without intervention, and test–retest reliability of .88. In contrast to the Burns (1985) study, there were no significant differences between graduated-prompt and mediational procedures in relation to the numbers of children who achieved a criterion level of independent performance.

These procedures and related research demonstrate that very young children can be assessed in a meaningful way with a dynamic format. These procedures differ from those applied to older populations in the decreased demands on attention, in the inclusion of manipulable materials, and in the more limited array of cognitive functions addressed.

5

Dynamic Assessment Research

In this chapter, the available research on dynamic assessment is presented and discussed. This review emphasizes work carried out in the United States, Canada, and Israel, with some reference to European studies that have been published in English. There is a significant body of European research that will be included in a soon-to-be-published text edited by Jan Hamers of The Netherlands (Hamers, in press). There is also a special issue of the *European Journal of Psychology of Education* (Vol. 5, No. 2, June 1990) that focuses on dynamic assessment. A copy of this special issue can be obtained from the publisher (the address is included in the "Resources" section of this book). Finally, Guthke (1982) provides an excellent and comprehensive overview of German-language research and instrument development. Information regarding specific instruments that have been developed in Germany can be obtained from the address included in the "Resources" section.

In this chapter, research specific to the primary dynamic assessment models (Feuerstein's and Budoff's) is discussed first. This is followed by a general discussion of research related to dynamic approaches to assessment of children's learning.

RESEARCH RELATED TO FEUERSTEIN'S LPAD

Less effort has been expended in researching the LPAD than has been directed at Instrumental Enrichment, Feuerstein's (1980) intervention

Some of the content of this chapter is based on a presentation to the International Conference on Cognitive Education, Mons, Belgium, July 1990.

curriculum. However, studies do exist, and data have been collected. The studies vary from focus on the instrumentation per se to applications of the LPAD to specialized populations (e.g., the deaf). Some of these studies involve individual administration, and some group administration. The specific LPAD tests included in the studies vary as well, but almost always include LPAD Variations I (matrix-type tasks), often Variations II, and the Representational Stencil Design Test (RSDT). When the group procedures have been used, the number of subjects has been impressively large. Since the number of studies is relatively small, each of those known to me is briefly mentioned here.

Three studies have dealt directly with the LPAD instrumentation. Watts (1985) investigated the frequency of occurrence of several of the cognitive deficiencies in relation to Raven's Standard Progressive Matrices. His subjects were 176 students in grades 3 through 9, with an age span of 9 years, 2 months through 15 years, 1 month. Watts operationalized cognitive deficiencies at the input and elaboration phases in terms of specific error choices on the Raven. He found that deficiencies at the elaboration phase occurred about twice as frequently as those at the input phase, and that occurrence of deficiencies did not vary with grade placement. The "use of limited sources of information," one of the deficiencies, accounted for most of the errors at the input phase. Elaborational deficiencies were strongly associated with error choices for students at all grade levels. Watts also analyzed high versus low scorers, and found that low scorers made significantly more irrelevant choices and showed more choices that indicated "lack of summative behavior" (another deficiency) than did high scorers.

Huberty and Cross (1988) compared two methods of scoring the RSDT: dichotomous (all or none; i.e., correct or not correct) versus nondichotomous (2 points for each item totally correct, and 1 point for correct design selection, but incorrect placement). Their subjects were 370 public school students in grades 7 and 8 in a large Midwestern urban area; IQs averaged 109.96, and achievement scores were at the upper end of the average range. Subjects were tested in groups of 15 to 25, and were provided with standard rather than "mediated" instructions. The alpha coefficient for the dichotomous method was .88, and for the nondichotomous method .92, with intercorrelation between the methods of .92. Split-half reliability for dichotomously scored protocols was .94, and for nondichotomously scored protocols .96. The scores were moderately but significantly correlated with IQ and all achievement variables (language, vocabulary, and math), and less closely related to achievement than to IQ. Factor analysis yielded different results for each scoring method. Analysis of the dichotomous scoring related primarily to item difficulty and yielded four factors. Analysis of the nondichotomous scoring yielded three factors, with the first factor accounting for a larger percentage of the total variance than the first factor of the dichotomous scoring method. The authors concluded that the nondichotomous scoring method was more "process"-oriented, more reliable, and more psychometrically valid.

Vaught and Haywood (1989) have reported results of an interjudge agreement study for ratings of the cognitive deficiencies on two LPAD tests: Variations I and RSDT. Two LPAD examiners administered these tests to four adolescents, and the videotaped procedures were sent to 10 "expert" judges for scoring. The list duplicated that of Feuerstein (1979), and the judges recorded yes–no evaluations regarding occurrence during the course of administration of each LPAD test; the judges also recorded intensity of mediation and response to mediation for each deficiency. Of the total 28 deficiencies, there was interrater agreement for all four subjects at 80% or above for 3 (blurred and sweeping perception, episodic grasp of reality, and egocentric communicational modalities). Another 4 deficiencies reached a level of agreement for all four subjects of 70% or above (failure to perceive the existence of and define a problem, trial-and-error responses, impaired communicative verbal tools, and impulsive acting-out behavior). Another 9 reached a level of agreement of 70% or above for three of the four subjects. Thus, a total of 16 deficiencies could be said to be scorable with at least "questionable" to high interrater agreement. This study also documented that the deficiencies on the Variations I instrument yielded much higher agreement (.77 coefficient) than ratings on the RSDT (.44). Also, the judges did not agree regarding intensity of mediation provided. Since I participated as a rater in this study, I can comment that even this level of modest agreement is impressive, in view of the fact that the definitions of the deficiencies were never really standardized across raters (each used his or her own interpretations); moreover, the adolescents who were assessed with the LPAD unpredictably turned out to be very capable performers, showing minimal evidence of deficiencies.

A good many data have been collected and some studies have been carried out by associates of the Jerusalem-based Hadassah-WIZO-Canada Research Institute, using the LPAD group procedures. Data reported in the basic text on the LPAD (Feuerstein, 1979) demonstrate significant gains in performance on the LPAD procedures (in some cases, individually administered), and, most importantly, changes in levels of performance that would not have been predicted by static tests. Numbers of adolescents who obtained static scores within the retarded ranges were able to demonstrate impressive responsiveness to mediation, and one group showed average-level scores on later results of the Israeli Army's IQ-like tests, statically administered.

Rand and Kaniel (1987) have reported a series of Israeli studies utilizing group administration procedures. In 1982, Rand administered the Variations I and II to a group of pupils in grades 4 through 7, from both "regular" and "culturally deprived" backgrounds. This study demonstrated significantly different performance between the two groups, as well as split-half coefficients from .82 to .89 for total scores, and subtest reliability coefficients ranging from moderate to high (all significant). In 1983, Rand studied 122 regular students in grade 5 with Variations I and II. This study yielded split-half coefficients for total scores ranging from .82 to .90; subtest coefficients were lower, but all were significant (alphas were at or beyond .01). That same year, Tzuriel and Rand administered Variations I and II to 595 culturally deprived and 799 regular students in grades 4 through 9. This study used three learning conditions during administration, varying in intensity of mediation: high, low, and no mediation. The Raven was administered before and after intervention, according to standard instructions. Both high- and low-mediation groups showed significant improvement in posttest Raven scores, compared to the no-mediation group, and the high-mediation group had significantly better posttest Raven scores than the low-mediation group. Subjects with initially high Raven scores were the least affected by the intensity of mediation.

Rand and Ben Shachar, in 1979, carried out a study with 337 pupils from grades 5 through 8. The Raven was administered as a pretest and posttest in standard format; the Variations I was administered to pupils in grades 5 and 6, and the Variations II was given to those in grades 7 and 8. Each grade was divided into two groups: mediation and no mediation. Mediated groups showed a significantly greater increase over nonmediated groups on posttest Raven scores. Finally, in 1979, Rand and Hoffman investigated 126 grade 9 and grade 10 students in a residential center; regular and low-functioning groups were compared. All students were administered the Primary Mental Abilities Test (PMA), as well as LPAD Variations II, RSDT, and Numerical Progressions. Despite the significant PMA differences, the groups did not show similar differences on the LPAD procedures. Classes were regrouped to reflect combined PMA and LPAD results. At the end of the school year, PMA and LPAD scores increased for both groups, and the initially lower subjects obtained scores on most measures significantly higher than those obtained on the pretests by the initially higher subjects. Pretest PMA differences disappeared for grade 10 pupils (but not grade 9 pupils) at posttest.

Luther and Wyatt's (1990) extensive study with low-SES high-school-level students in North York, Ontario, provides evidence for both concurrent and predictive validity of the group-administered LPAD. These researchers found the LPAD to correlate significantly with WISC/WAIS-R IQ, as well as with grades in school (the correlation was stronger with grades than with IQ). Students with IQs below 60 did not do well on the LPAD, but many students with IQs in the 70s did well both on the LPAD and academically (in their special needs schools). Finally, their results showed no relationship between scores on the WAIS-R Similarities subtest (administered in the standardized way) and scores of a standardized reading comprehension test, but a highly positive correlation between the enriched Similarities (incorporated into the LPAD) and reading comprehension.

Several studies of the LPAD have been carried out with specialized populations, including the deaf, the gifted, and the learning-disabled. Huberty and Koller (1984) used the RSDT with deaf and hearing students in grades 7 and 8. The hearing group included 24 boys and 16 girls, with an average age of 12 years, 11 months; the deaf subjects included 14 boys and 14 girls, with an average age of 12 to 15 years. In the case of hearing subjects, the authors selected high and low achievers in terms of levels at the top and bottom 25% on the Stanford Achievement Tests (SAT); in the case of the deaf subjects, high achievers were defined as above the 65th percentile and low achievers as below the 35th percentile on the SAT norms. There were no significant differences between hearing and deaf subjects in achievement. All subjects were randomly assigned to training and nontraining groups. A partial (nondichotomous) scoring method was used for the RSDT. Only the achievement levels were associated with RSDT pretest scores for both groups. Achievement, training, and hearing status all showed significant effects on posttest scores; high achievers did better, and trained subjects did better. Training helped low achievers and not high achievers to improve. Trained low achievers did as well as trained high achievers, and there were no differences between deaf and hearing subjects.

Katz and Buchholz (1984) reported a case study of a 14-year-old deaf girl with dull-normal IQ. This girl was selected because she appeared to her teachers to be brighter than her IQ score indicated. Seven LPAD tests were administered over a 6-week period, for a total of over 30 hours. The authors described the girl's responses in terms of strengths and weaknesses, progress on tasks, and examples of mediations employed.

Keane and Kretschmer (1987) investigated the effectiveness of mediation with six LPAD tests in a deaf population. These subjects included 45 profoundly deaf children between the ages of 10 and 11 years, with low-average IQs. There were three groups: an experimental group that received mediation, a comparison control group that received elaborated feedback, and a no-treatment control group. Pre- and postintervention instruments included the nonverbal portion of the Cognitive Abilities Test and the Kohs Blocks Design Test. The mediated group performed significantly better than either control group on all LPAD tasks except Associated Recall (a task that was administered the same way to all groups, thereby serving an an internal control). On Organization of Dots and Plateaux, the elaborated-feedback group performed better than the no-treatment control. In terms of effects on the Cognitive Abilities Test, both the mediated and elaborated-feedback groups did better than the no-treatment controls, but there was no difference between the mediated and elaborated-feedback groups on this measure. On the Kohs, only the mediated group showed an increase in the number of designs successfully completed and a decrease in the number of trials needed for successful completion.

Skuy, Kaniel, and Tzuriel (1988) have reported a study in which the group LPAD was used to identify gifted students from a low-SES population in Israel. All the students from 35 classes in five Israeli primary schools (grades 4 through 6, and ages 9 through 11) were included in the study, with a total *n* of 1,041. Most of the pupils were native-born Jewish children of parents who immigrated from Arab countries. On the basis of teacher identification and grades, a group of students achieving at the top of their class was selected; these subjects constituted group 1. Nonselected students constituted group 2. All students were assessed with the LPAD group measures (Verbal Analogies, Organizer, Variations I) for 15 hours of testing over a 3-week period. Prior to administration of the LPAD tests, the students took an Israeli IQ test, based on the WISC Verbal subtests; the Raven was administered as a pretest and posttest. Significant differences resulted between groups 1 and 2 on all pretests; however, group 1's Raven scores were in the superior range (90th percentile), whereas the Raven scores for group 2 were average (50th percentile). Posttest scores for the Raven and Organizer were significantly higher for both groups; this was not so for Verbal Analogies. Group 1 showed the most change on the Organizer.

Finally, two publications report results of the use of LPAD procedures with learning-disabled students. Samuels, Tzuriel, and Malloy-Miller (1989) review the work conducted with the LPAD at The Learning Centre in Calgary, Alberta, affiliated with the University of Calgary. From their experience in using the LPAD with adults, the authors concluded that it was most useful (1) with adults with low literacy and some social adjustment problems, and (2) with adults with good literacy and poor social–emotional adjustment. They found it less useful with adults with very specific learning disabilities. The useful aspect of the LPAD was ascribed to the supportive examiner–client relationship, which was especially helpful to clients who were fearful of tests and had low self-esteem.

Samuels et al. (1989) also report a study carried out in 1987 with children with learning difficulties. In this study, examiner agreement regarding ratings of cognitive deficiencies was 87.6%, and agreement regarding ratings of mediation was 91.6%. This study compared children classified as mildly retarded, as learning-disabled with and without attention deficits, and as normal (the control group). On Organization of Dots, the retarded scored lower than all other groups, with no significant differences among other groups; the retarded group required more time to complete the test phase. On the Raven, the retarded scored lower, with no differences among the other groups. This was essentially the pattern on all the measures, with the order of performance showing the normals as scoring highest, the learning-disabled groups achieving intermediate scores, and the retarded scoring lowest. The authors found the retarded group in general to respond to mediation, but to respond more slowly and at a lower level. On the Organizer, the retarded performed as well as the learning-disabled groups; the learning-disabled had the most difficulty with the Orga-nizer. Normals performed best on all measures, and the learning-disabled with attention deficits had consistently more difficulty than either the normals or the learning-disabled without attention deficits. Regarding ratings of deficiencies, Samuels et al. found differences in degree rather than in kind between groups; the retarded had the most, and the normals the least. The most frequently used mediational behaviors for all groups were focusing, prompting, promoting meta-cognitive awareness, teaching rules and strategies, and mediation of competence. Although level of performance could have been predicted by WISC-R IQ for all groups, IQ was not an effective discriminator between the two learning-disabled groups; these two groups did, however, show consistent LPAD differences, with attention deficit pupils requiring more mediation and manifesting more deficiencies. Furthermore, the IQ scores would not have been able to predict the responsiveness of the retarded group to mediation.

Finally, Skuy, Archer, and Roth (1987) have reported a case study in which the LPAD was used with an 11-year-old girl diagnosed as learning-disabled. The LPAD was administered over a 3-month period on a weekly basis for 16 sessions; this included testing as well as intervention that addressed content areas of math and geography.

However, postintervention testing did not include transfer of effects to either math or geography. Intervention strategies emphasized meta-cognitive awareness, planning, self-regulation, competence, and meaning. The girl showed improvement on all measures, with the exceptions of section E on the Raven and the WISC-R Block Design. Her total Raven percentile increased from 85th to 95th, and her scores on the WISC-R Object Assembly and Picture Arrangement subtests improved as well. The authors see this study as providing insights into intervention needs and strategies.

To summarize, studies such as those described in this section are beginning to provide needed information regarding the psychometric properties, as well as applications, of the LPAD. So far, there are indications of adequate intratest consistency, fair to moderate inter-rater agreement, and stronger evidence regarding concurrent and predictive validity of some of the instruments. Mediation does seem to produce differences in performance, and its effects appear stronger for initially low performers. Nondichotomous scoring appears more sensitive, reliable, and valid than dichotomous scoring, when there is a choice. Also, more precise and well-supported descriptions of the intervention behaviors that appear most useful and effective, as well as the cognitive functions and deficiencies that relate most strongly to overall performance, are beginning to become available.

RESEARCH RELATED TO BUDOFF'S PROCEDURES

Research studies concerning psychometric properties of Budoff's procedures have already been reviewed in Chapter 3. In this section, research utilizing his procedures to explore "learning potential" as a concept is presented.

Some general results of Budoff and associates' research include typical findings of a strong relationship between the learning potential assessment (LPA) measures and WISC Performance IQ. Also, with the exception of the Picture Word Game (PWG), the procedures appear to minimize effects of race and SES. The research has also demonstrated that the improvements found can be attributed to the training procedure employed and not to practice; although practice effects have at times been found, these tend to be exceeded by training effects (Budoff, 1987a).

Another question of interest is the extent to which results on LPA measures correlate with each other (i.e., how consistent performance is across LPA measures). Some evidence regarding this is available in

Babad and Bashi (1975), who found a correlation of .38 between the Raven Learning Potential Test (RLPT) and Series Learning Potential Test (SLPT) as pretests, and .50 between them as posttests. Their subjects were 200 Israeli sixth-grade students.

A number of researchers have incorporated Budoff's approach into their studies, with mixed results. Sewell and Severson (1974), researching the relationships among IQ, diagnostic teaching, and the RLPT with 62 black first-grade children, found that the RLPT results had as strong a relationship as IQ with reading, and a stronger relationship than IQ with arithmetic. The three conditions (feedback, social praise, and tangible reinforcement) of diagnostic teaching had the strongest relationship with both achievement measures. The pretest of the RLPT showed minimal relationship with achievement, while both RLPT posttest and gain scores showed a relationship with achievement equal to that of IQ. The RLPT scores were also shown to contribute to achievement independently of IQ.

Sewell (1979) also investigated the differential predictive value of IQ and LPA for black and white first-graders. Budoff's RLPT was used. For combined groups, the RLPT pretest was as good a predictor of achievement as IQ, whereas the RLPT posttest exceeded IQ in predicting both reading and math (.41 vs. .54 for reading, and .52 vs. .63 for math). IQ was a more consistently reliable predictor of achievement for blacks than for whites. However, in a stepwise regression analysis, the RLPT posttest was the only significant contributor to achievement prediction for blacks, and the only significant contributor to total achievement prediction for both whites and blacks; IQ did not contribute significantly for either group.

Using an older (third-grade), mixed-SES sample, Popoff-Walker (1982) assessed the relative responsiveness of normally functioning and EMR students to practice versus training on the RLPT, and researched the relative effects of SES and adaptive behavior as well. The author found both IQ groups to profit from training, with non-EMRs showing more gain than EMRs. On the RLPT, training was associated with more score improvement than practice, but this did not reach significance. EMRs' scores changed only in response to practice or training; non-EMRs' scores improved even without these conditions, although they showed greater improvement with the interventions of practice or training. Although this study showed that the RLPT scores of the EMRs never reached the pretest levels of the non-EMRs, some important qualifications need to be made. There was a seeming lack of independence of SES and IQ for many of the analyses, and Popoff-Walker pointed out that a number of subjects had neurologically based deficits; these deficits would be less likely to respond to short interventions such as the 45-minute training sessions offered in this study. Also, there were no separate analyses offered for EMR subjects with and without normal adaptive behavior scores, although the author pointed out that adaptive behavior was not a good predictor of learning potential. Finally, the point was made that a more individualized training procedure might have had a greater chance of effectiveness with the EMR children.

Wurtz, Sewell, and Manni (1985) used the RLPT as a criterion measure against which to compare the effectiveness of Estimated Learning Potential (ELP; derived from the System of Multicultural Pluralistic Assessment [SOMPA]) and WISC-R IQs. The rationale of a learning procedure rather than achievement scores as a criterion measure addresses the similarity of IQ and achievement tests on such dimensions as cultural loading. These two measures can also be equated in terms of static outcomes; the authors note the fact that IQ tests have been validated in terms of achievement scores, with items and subtests selected and therefore evaluated in terms of the extent to which they are associated with achievement. The Wurtz et al. study investigated the relationship of ELP and IQ to RLPT scores for 63 low-SES, black and white, 10-year-old, urban EMR students. Blacks differed from whites in their RLPT pretest and posttest scores, but not in their ELPs or IQs. ELPs and IQs for both blacks and whites did not differ in terms of prediction of RLPT posttest scores. Furthermore, neither IQ nor ELP correlated significantly with achievement for the total group, and IQ significantly correlated with achievement only for whites. Although this point is not discussed in the article, it is also of interest to note from the analysis of one of the tables that correlations between IQ and RLPT were stronger for pretests than for posttests (significance not determined); that the relationship with RLPT was even stronger in for ELP than for IQ; and that the RLPT posttest (not the pretest) correlated significantly with reading, but only for whites. The fact of reduced correlation of IQ with pretests versus posttests supports the interpretation that "response to intervention" may be a phenomenon not entirely coincident with IQ.

Thus, although these studies are mixed in their provision of evidence supporting learning potential as an effective predictor of the school functioning of low-SES black or EMR students, the studies also do not support the effectiveness of IQ as a meaningful predictor of the school success of these students. In some cases, the RLPT posttest was as good a predictor as IQ.

RESEARCH RELATED TO THE DYNAMIC
ASSESSMENT MODEL IN GENERAL

Research on the topic of dynamic assessment has consistently supported at least six conclusions:

First, mediation is associated with improved performance on a
variety of tasks for a variety of learners.

Second, practice alone does not account for these effects, at least not
on complex learning tasks.

Third, two of the most powerful components within this mediational
effect seem to be verbalization and elaborated feedback, with the
feedback including information about the correctness of the performance that conveys a rationale for, and the principles of, task solution.

Fourth, mediated interventions seem to be associated with the
greatest degree of improvement for lower-functioning students, although positive effects for other groups have also been demonstrated.

Fifth, IQ outpredicts learning indicators primarily when the criteria
involve other static scores. When the criteria involve process dimensions, dynamic approaches do at least as well as, and often better than,
IQ.

Sixth, dynamic assessment results make a significant and independent contribution to achievement variance, above and beyond IQ.

The research that has generated these conclusions is now briefly
reviewed.

1. Mediation Is Associated with Improved Performance   Burns
(1985) and Burns, Vye, Bransford, Delclos, and Ogan (1987) demonstrated that graduated-prompt intervention and mediated intervention
were both superior to static test performance on a modified stencil
design activity. Mediated intervention in the Burns (1985) study was
superior to both static and graduated-prompt intervention on a transfer
task. Studies with the LPAD, especially those conducted with the group
procedures by researchers such as Kaniel, Tzuriel, and Skuy, have
provided consistent evidence of the positive effects of mediation. Paour
(in press) has also demonstrated positive effects with young French
children, using his procedure.

2. Practice Alone Does Not Account for These Effects   The
limited effectiveness of practice alone was evident in the research of
Rohwer (1971), when he found that only his high-SES subjects were
able to profit from practice, while his low-SES subjects required
training in what he called "elaborative skills" (which included imagery,

verbal mediation, and rehearsal strategies). In her study of 43 preschool Canadian children with special needs, Missiuna (1986) found lack of improvement in the scores of her "practice-only" group, using the Tzuriel and Klein (1985) Children's Analogical Test of Modifiability (CATM) procedure. Children receiving mediational intervention outperformed both the practice and the instructional intervention groups.

In a 1987 study using the LPAD procedures with deaf students, Keane and Kretschmer (1987) reported a lack of practice effects, with superiority of the mediated group over both the elaborated-feedback and practice-only groups. Embretson (1987), in a study of college students working on a spatial concept task, found some improvement in the performance of her practice group, but not to the extent of those receiving intervention. Studies utilizing LPAD instruments have also been successful in ruling in the positive effects of mediation, while ruling out practice effects. This is evident, for example, in the work of Kaniel, Tzuriel, Feuerstein, Ben-Shachar, and Eitan (1989) with 306 immigrant Ethiopian adolescents in Israel. And, finally, in two recent doctoral dissertations (Reinharth, 1989; Thomas, 1984) using the Preschool Learning Assessment Device (see Part III of this book), the mediated groups significantly outperformed the practice groups.

It thus appears to be a robust finding across a variety of ages with a variety of materials and domains that more than practice is necessary to induce improved performance, especially for lower-functioning and low-SES children. In some cases, higher-functioning children were more able to profit from unmediated practice.

Bortner and Birch (1969) demonstrated many years ago that children often possess more capacity than is evident in their observed performance. They suggested, even before the days of awareness of dynamic assessment procedures, that higher levels of performance could be elicited if researchers could find a way to access them. For example, the apparent inability of very young children to determine which of two groups of candy has "more," in a traditionally presented Piagetian task, is easily and accurately solved when the question is changed to "Which would you like to eat?" From their own research and their review of others' research, Bortner and Birch concluded:

> Possessed concepts and skills, and particular conceptual abilities, as well as levels of learning, when manifested in performance, all reflect the interaction between possessed potentialities and the particular conditions of training and task demands. Glaring differences occur in the estimates of potential when meaningful alterations are made in the conditions of performance. (p. 742)

**3. Two of the Most Powerful Components Seem to Be Verbaliza-
tion and Elaborated Feedback**   Most of the evidence for the power
of verbalization and elaborated feedback derives from the studies of
Carlson and Wiedl and their collaborators (e.g., Carlson & Wiedl,
1980; Cormier, Carlson, & Das, no date). Keane and Kretschmer
(1987) found exactly the same results with their deaf children; Collins,
Carnine, and Gersten (1987) report similar results using computer-
assisted instruction with learning-disabled and remedial high school
students; and Symons and Vye (1986) demonstrated the greater
effectiveness of conditions including elaborated feedback with their
4-year-old, normally functioning Canadian children. It is important to
point out that the elaborated-feedback condition of these studies
included not only information about correctness of performance, but
statement of the general principle involved in problem solution. Such
evidence takes us well beyond behavioristic into cognitive explanations
of learning. In their attempts to understand the mechanism of this
phenomenon, Bethge, Carlson, and Wiedl (1982) showed that the
verbalization and elaborated-feedback conditions led to increases in
planful behavior in the learner, as well as to decreased anxiety.

**4. Mediated Interventions Seem to Result in Most Improvement
for Lower-Functioning Students**   Although the prediction of future
performance raises complex issues, not the least of which has to do with
criterion adequacy, a study by Babad and Bashi (1975) at Budoff's
research institute suggested that IQ appeared to be a better predictor of
future static achievement of students whose families were characterized
by higher levels of education, whereas LPA procedures provided better
predictions for students from families with lower educational backgrounds. However, when the criterion measure changed from static
achievement to a more process-oriented curriculum-based test, the
LPA procedures were the best predictors for both groups. In their
multiple-regression analysis, the LPA posttest scores far outpredicted
both IQ and standardized achievement tests in relation to the criterion
of a curriculum-based test.

In another study, Babad and Budoff (1974) again obtained results
suggesting that their EMR and low-normal to average, low-SES
subjects profited the most from learning potential training, whereas IQ
was the better predictor of static achievement for their above-average
group.

Campione and Brown (1990) conclude from their many studies that
"the weaker the student, the more the need for detailed and explicit
instruction" (p. 144). They also found their weak students very
reluctant to employ learned strategies in new situations. They were able

to help them overcome this reluctance with extensive practice, but it was transfer that continued to be the most reliable discriminator between their retarded and nonretarded groups.

Also, studies by both Scrofani, Suziedelis, and Shore (1975) and Tzuriel (1989) found that low-SES subjects profited the most from the interventions offered, despite differences in tasks, types of interventions, and age groups. However, contrary evidence is offered by Popoff-Walker (1982), who compared normal third-grade achievers with low-functioning EMR subjects, using Budoff's RLPT. In this case, the nonretarded children profited the most from the training, although the EMR children did improve.

5. IQ Outpredicts Learning Indicators Primarily When the Criteria Involve Other Static Scores Budoff, Meskin, and Harrison (1971) found that when their criterion was progress in an electricity unit, the initial pretest distinctions between their regular and special education subjects disappeared on the posttests; however, the two groups remained distinguishable in their ability to provide causal explanations for problems they were able to solve nonverbally.

Camp (1973), in her study of severely dyslexic 9- to 13-year-olds participating in a tutorial program, found significant correlations between psychometric tests, but not between these tests and learning rate. And Campione and Brown (1990), in a summary of studies from their laboratory, report research by Bryant with 4- and 5-year-old children that found dynamic assessment scores to be better predictors of residualized gain than static IQ (WPPSI and Raven).

Occasionally, however, learning ability will even provide a better prediction of static achievement than IQ. For example, Hegarty (1988), using his National Foundation for Educational Research (NFER) Test of Children's Learning Ability (Hegarty, 1979), described a study conducted with Lewis in 1978 with 420 immigrant 7-year-olds in England; they compared IQ based on a short form of the WISC with achievement tests given 1 year later. They found learning ability to be a better predictor of achievement than WISC IQ.

6. Dynamic Assessment Results Make a Significant and Independent Contribution to Achievement Variance, above and beyond IQ Bransford, Delclos, Vye, Burns, and Hasselbring (1986), in their report to the American Psychological Association (APA) Subcommittee on Testing and Special Education, review their studies demonstrating that a substantial percentage of children within each of three McCarthy Scales score subgroups were able to reach a criterion level on a stencil design task. Although the percentage of children reaching criterion increased with an increase in McCarthy GCI, 36% of even the lowest group (GCIs of 37–52) reached criterion. Day and Hall (1987) reported their research showing wide variability in initial learning of children obtaining IQs in the retarded ranges, and found that these children were among both the fastest and the slowest in their dynamic assessment performance. Day and Hall also reported that their dynamic assessment results accounted for a significant amount of variance above and beyond IQ in predicting transfer and learning. Hamilton and Budoff (1974), with 40 institutionalized mentally retarded subjects between the ages of 12 and 22 and Peabody Picture Vocabulary Test IQs ranging from below 10 to 51, found both their high and low groups to profit from the training. They also found a significant relationship between "gainer" versus "nongainer" status and teacher ratings, and their results documented a significant relationship of IQ to the learning potential pretest scores, but not the posttest results.

And, finally, Speece, Cooper, and Kibler (1989) carried out a regression analysis of the degree of contribution of several measures to posttest performance on their dynamic assessment procedure, used with 192 first-grade children. They found that number of prompts needed during the training phase accounted for a small but significant proportion of the variance, above and beyond that contributed by other measures.

There are also some studies that are not easily categorized but that introduce some important dimensions of dynamic assessment research. For example, Vye, Burns, Delclos, and Bransford (1987) have documented difficulty with cross-domain transfer, using dynamic assessment procedures. And Delclos, Burns, and Kulewicz (1987) demonstrated the positive effects of viewing dynamic versus static assessment on teachers' stated expectations of student performance.

6

Issues and Concluding Remarks

The reader has now been introduced to the prevailing ideas and procedures of dynamic assessment. Although it is still in its developing stages, the field is no longer in a neonatal phase, and there is a great deal of activity and energy being devoted to applying the basic concepts of modifiability, process, and linkage to instructional variables. It has been somewhat easier to develop new procedures than to investigate some of the basic questions and issues associated not only with the dynamic assessment model, but with assessment in general. Perhaps one of the major contributions of dynamic assessment has been to raise questions and refocus research attention on issues that many feel are of more concern than those that have been the focus of so much research literature. It is relatively easy to generate data addressing traditional concepts of reliability and validity. It is considerably more difficult to study issues of quality, meaning, and process, all closely associated with dynamic assessment.

QUESTIONS AND ISSUES FOR THE FUTURE

I have recently been in the position of being requested to perform dynamic assessments by parents of handicapped children. These parents are all highly informed and articulate, have all been exposed to traditional psychometrics, and have found the information wanting. They do not deny the facts of low levels of performance in their children, but follow these conclusions with remarks such as these: "So what? What does that tell me that is meaningful about my child?" or

"When my child is reassessed, all I can find out is another IQ score. How does this help me help my child?" Conducting these assessments has made it clear how limited the usefulness of the quantitative information can be. If the focus were solely on scores and score changes, there would be little to say except to confirm that such a child is indeed a low-level performer. By contrast, the focus on the process and intervention components in dynamic assessment generates a great deal of information and leaves the parents with the feeling that they have learned something meaningful. Also, when the parents are able to be present during the course of the assessment, they find it particularly helpful to reinforce and guide their own interactions with their child.

The dilemma, however, remains: How do we "measure" this? If we strive to be scientific and to gain credibility for dynamic assessment within the social sciences, there needs to be some way to demonstrate effects and effectiveness. In order to do this, we have to pose questions in ways that facilitate research and adequately reflect the nature of the dynamic assessment process. We also need to rethink many of our old assumptions, and to realize, first of all, that these are assumptions and not established facts. For example, we have assumed intelligence to be a stable trait, and have designed tests and experiments to reflect this assumption. It is an assumption, not necessarily a fact. When it is assumed that intelligence is stable, items on tests are then thrown out when they fail to demonstrate this stability, and tests are dismissed as defective when they fail to show high test–retest stability. We are then engaged in designing a world that supports our assumptions. The potential effects of such assumptions and the research methodology related to them were pointed out by Estes (1981) when he attributed the history of low correlations between learning and intelligence to dif-fering methods of measurement. Estes observed that studies of intelli-gence have typically relied on correlational methods, whereas studies of learning have relied on experimental designs. Furthermore, intelli-gence tests assess performance over a short period of time and are deliberately designed to reduce the effects of learning, whereas learning ability measures require long periods of time in order to show effects. Therefore, it is possible that the low correlations reflect "variations in context rather than independence of the abilities" (p. 13).

Dynamic assessment and the cognitive education field to which it relates are based on an assumption that intelligence is modifiable. The challenge, then, is to find the means for improving cognitive function-ing. This does not require the additional assumption that all individuals are infinitely modifiable, or that, given appropriate interventions, all individuals have the potential for genius. However, it does require an open-mindedness in regard to the possibility that a static level-of-performance score may not indicate just how much an individual can change. This suggests a need to modify definitions of intelligence to include "learning ability" or "responsivity to intervention." The research that has been generated has documented that dynamic assessment procedures do account for additional variance even in relation to static achievement scores, and that individuals who appear similar in terms of their psychometric performance may look very different in terms of their responses to learning ability procedures. There are even instances when dynamic assessment results outpredict IQ. Clearly, dynamic assessment measures, although correlated with IQ, are tapping something quite different, and this "different" quality appears relevant to the child's functioning in a learning situation. Haywood, Filler, Shifman, and Chatalanet (1975) expressed related thoughts when they wrote:

> Obviously, the narrower the band of predicted events, the greater the success of the predictive instrument. When used to predict relative standing on academic achievement, traditional intelligence tests are moderately successful, their scores being associated with as much as 50 percent of the variance in subsequent achievement measures. Such a success rate is of considerable academic interest, unless one is concerned with the other 50 percent of the variance. (pp. 98–99)

Clearly, those interested in dynamic assessment and in cognitive education in general are interested in the other 50% of the variance.

What we need to do now is to be careful in our descriptions to note which type of dynamic assessment procedure relates to which type of criterion. We must avoid lumping all procedures under the one term and then attributing research findings to a generic concept of "dynamic assessment." The procedures differ considerably in regard to content domains, sequencing of tasks, standardization, time involvement, and populations involved. Any conclusions need to be discussed in relation to these and other variables.

The issue of criteria is one that presents ongoing difficulty and challenge in any discussion of dynamic assessment. Validity studies require a criterion of comparison, whether for concurrent, predictive, or construct purposes. Researchers have used a variety of criteria, including static achievement scores, gain scores, and learning curves. McClelland (1973) expressed the issue very poignantly:

> The games people are required to play on aptitude tests are similar to the games teachers require in the classroom. . . . So it is scarcely surprising that aptitude test scores are correlated highly with grades in school. . . .

Defenders of intelligence testing . . . often seem to be suggesting that
this is the only kind of validity necessary. . . . Researchers have in fact
had great difficulty demonstrating that grades in school are related to
any other behavior of importance—other than doing well on aptitude
tests. (pp. 1–2)

McClelland goes on to note:

It is difficult, if not impossible, to find a human characteristic that
cannot be modified by training or experience. . . . To the traditional
intelligence tester this fact has been something of a nuisance because he
has been searching for some unmodifiable, unfakable index of innate
mental capacity. (p. 8)

Feuerstein (1979) suggested that the only valid criterion for a
dynamic assessment procedure is the child's responsiveness to instruction based upon the results of the assessment. This makes a great deal
of sense. First of all, the only meaningful criterion for process as an
independent variable would be process as a dependent variable.
Although it is fortuitous when significant correlations occur in relation
to static criteria, it is not a basis for negative evaluation of the process
assessment instrument when this does not occur. If we say that the
information generated from dynamic assessment concerns responsiveness to instruction, then this procedure is only fairly evaluated in
relation to a "responsiveness" indicator. However, as important as this
observation is, the second portion of Feuerstein's observation is even
more critical and more often overlooked: namely, that the intervention
should be based on the results of the assessment. It is under these
conditions that the child's responsiveness becomes meaningful. If I, as
a diagnostic specialist, assess the child and make recommendations
derived from my assessment, and these are not implemented, then the
usefulness of my assessment cannot be determined (except, perhaps, in
terms of the teacher's judgment regarding the utility of the assessment).
    The issue of transfer is of particular interest. Dynamic assessment
has been more successful in demonstrating responsiveness to intervention than in inducing successful transfer; yet transfer has been shown
to be the best discriminator between retarded and nonretarded performers. The question of the appropriateness of attempting induction
of transfer has not really been posed and considered. Dynamic
assessment is, after all, assessment, and not the learning situation itself.
Assessment is, by definition, a sample of behavior. When dynamic
assessment is used for diagnostic purposes, it may not be realistic to
expect transfer effects. On the other hand, evidence of ability to

transfer may be a useful index of higher potential in an otherwise low-level performer. Transfer may be most relevantly included when dynamic assessment is used to check and monitor mastery within domains of achievement, as has been suggested by Campione and Brown (1990); in this case, readiness to move to the next learning step may be preceded by assessment of transfer as an indicator of mastery. In any case, the appropriateness of including a transfer component needs careful consideration and discussion.

Dynamic assessment deals with the very essence of learning: how to restructure thinking; how to pass on knowledge from expert to novice; how to induce capabilities for independent problem solution. There are issues regarding determination of what a child knows and can do, and of how to move him from that point *a* to point *b*. We need increased consensus regarding the process characteristics of the learner and the effective components of mediation — those that are general, and those that are domain-specific. We seem to agree regarding the general objective of inducing self-regulating, efficient, active, and strategic learning in a broad array of domains. It is not the task of dynamic assessment to determine the domains; these need to reflect the cultur-ally determined decisions of the society in which the learner is embedded, and these may be expected to vary over time even within a culture. It is the task of dynamic assessment to try to uncover the nature of the learner, and to increase the match between this nature and the outcomes required for survival and success within the learner's culture. Dynamic assessment, as developed, has been primarily con-cerned with improving the child's ability to function within a Western, technologically oriented society; it has special value, in conjunction with cognitive education, for children whose early experiences fail to prepare them to cope adequately with the demands of such a culture.

CRITERIA FOR EVALUATING DYNAMIC ASSESSMENT

Dynamic assessment, like any form of assessment, needs criteria by which to be evaluated. I have spent time here criticizing existing bases of evaluation, suggesting that they are not appropriate when applied to the dynamic assessment model. It is usually less difficult to criticize than to propose solutions. In the case of dynamic assessment, it is likewise easier to say what is wrong with existing criteria of evaluation than to propose criteria that may be deemed more useful and effective. It seems appropriate at this point to pose the question of what constitutes a "good" dynamic assessment. Are there any generalizable criteria, given the diversity of approaches? On the basis of the information available, some broad criteria are suggested; these are offered here as starting points, with expectations of changes and modifications as experience increases. Dynamic assessment procedures are viewed as needing to respond to the following questions:

1. *What is the underlying theory of intelligence?* Authors of psychometric approaches to measurement of intelligence have become increasingly theory-conscious, realizing the importance of explicitly stating the basis for derivation of their procedures. Without a theory, it is very difficult to evaluate the relevance and information value of the procedure. It is the theory that generates the processes to be addressed by the assessment. Without a theory, there is no answer to these questions: Why these items? Why these particular processes? Why this means of assessment? Why this test?

2. *What are the processes addressed in the learner?* Dynamic assessment is, by definition, process-oriented. These processes flow directly from the underlying theories. It is necessary to know what to look for in the learner in order to derive conclusions about her functioning. These processes should reflect what is known about "good learners."

3. *What are the principles for examiner interaction, and how do these relate to instructional criteria?* There needs to be a basis for guiding examiner behavior and for deriving conclusions generated by these behaviors. This basis needs to reflect what is known about "good instruction," since the purpose of the assessment is to provide a sample of an optimal instructional interaction.

4. *Does the information generated from the assessment lead to improved learner functioning within the classroom?* The information generated should include descriptions of the learner's responsiveness, characteristics of processing, and effective (and ineffective) interventions. These need to be relevant to classroom instructional variables and to be utilizable by a reasonably well-trained teacher who does incorporate the assessment recommendations into instruction (who indeed, in some cases, may be the assessor). This criterion is as relevant to psychometric assessment as to dynamic assessment, but has rarely if ever been applied.

5. *Would independent, equally well-trained assessors derive similar conclusions and types of recommendations from the assessment?* Although it would be unlikely for two individuals to interact in exactly the same way when conducting a dynamic assessment, particularly of the unstandardized variety, it should be demonstrable that similar or "ballpark" conclusions about the learner can be derived. Consumers need to be assured that the results of the assessment are not entirely examiner-dependent, and that meaningful information about a child can result.

6. *Is the procedure teachable?* Dynamic assessment is useful only to the extent that it is used. Assessors need to be able to master the concepts

and procedures, which differ considerably from what is traditionally taught. Procedures need to be designed and explained with such dissemination potential in mind. On the other hand, the implementation of dynamic assessment needs to be in the hands of professionals who have a thorough and profound understanding of child development, assessment theory, educational interventions, and clinical interaction. In the most clinical format, these procedures are very difficult because the specialist has to think and react extemporaneously; the *t*'s are not crossed, and the *i*'s are not dotted; there is no list of questions to ask or selection of responses to consider as correct.

7. *Can the procedure be administered within a "reasonable" period of time?* What is "reasonable" will vary considerably from situation to situation, and the constant quest for "quick fixes" needs to be resisted in favor of quality; clearly, however, efficiency and utility are issues for assessors who have large caseloads and who may be using a variety of assessment procedures. Attention needs to be paid to establishing the time needed to generate the necessary information, and then to advocating for having this time allotted. The array of dynamic assessment procedures currently available is applicable under a variety of conditions, with some more appropriate for screening, some for group administration, some for monitoring, and others for in-depth and comprehensive diagnostic exploration.

Collins (1990) brings to focus the often insidious effect that testing can have on education. Although some may think that testing is a background to education and reflects the goals of education, it can often be the other way around: "Testing affects what is taught in the schools. . . . [Tests] become the standards by which school systems, teachers, and students are judged. They unconsciously dictate what students should learn" (p. 75).

In fact, we might more accurately determine the objectives of education by reviewing its tests than by reviewing its curricula. If this is so, concern with testing and assessment is far from trivial: We need to ask what we want our schools to teach, and to examine the instruments of assessment to see whether these objectives are reflected. Collins offers his list of "shoulds":

1. Tests should emphasize learning and thinking . . . in particular, problem-solving strategies . . . , self-regulatory or monitoring strategies, and learning strategies. . . .
2. Tests should require generation as well as selection. . . .
3. Tests should be integral to learning. . . .
4. Tests should serve multiple purposes . . . (a) motivating students to study and directing that study to certain topics or issues; (b) diagnosing what difficulties students are having and selecting what they

should study next; (c) placing students in classes, grades, schools, and jobs; (d) reporting to students, teachers, and parents on the progress a student has made; and (e) evaluating how well a teacher, school, or school system is doing vis à vis other teachers, schools and systems. . . .

    5. Tests should be valid with respect to all their purposes. (pp. 78–79)

If these are taken as criteria for evaluation of an assessment program, then dynamic assessment would seem to be a necessary addition to the existing repertory of psychometric, developmental, and criterion-referenced approaches.

One of the problems obstructing incorporation of dynamic assessment into courses that train assessors is the perception of a poor fit between the objectives of the assessment and of the educational settings of the assessors (Lidz, in press-b). The problem is not that the information generated by the assessment is viewed as irrelevant, but that the bill-paying consumers (administrators and legislators, not teachers) value quantity and speed, and not necessarily quality. If we analyze what is valued in education in terms of the criterion of what is assessed by the tests, the results suggest product orientation and rote memorization. Little attention is paid to approaches to problem solving, or to analysis of errors or metacognition, in our traditional and prevailing assessment procedures; in fact, there is little attention to the process of attention. How, then, can we expect these objectives to infiltrate the educational establishment? Conversely, if they do not become educational objectives, there is no rationale for their inclusion in assessments. Glaser (1981) reflects this observation when he says:

> There is little empirically derived and conceptually understood relationship between test score information and specific instructional activity. . . . I see little significant progress . . . unless more flexible environments are introduced in school systems . . . [that] would permit differential instructional practices that could be coordinated with useful diagnostic assessment so that the testing and the teaching become integral events. (pp. 924–925)

CONCLUDING REMARKS

When I was in graduate school studying psychometrics and individual assessment, Anastasi, Cronbach, and Tyler—the authors of the major texts in the field—were among the psychometric giants. These foundation builders have become increasingly discontented with traditional psychometric approaches to assessment. For example, Anastasi (1981) observes:

The concept [of intelligence] that is now emerging differs in several important ways from the earlier concept of intelligence that prevailed from the turn of the century to the 1930s, and that still survives in popular discussions of intelligence, intelligence testing, and that particular horror, the IQ. . . . Intelligence tests are [now] seen as measures of what the individual has learned to do and what he or she knows at the time. Tests can serve a predictive function only insofar as they indicate to what extent the individual has acquired the prerequisite skills and knowledge for a designated criterion performance. What persons can accomplish in the future depends not only on their present intellectual status, as assessed by the test, but also on their subsequent experiences.

Furthermore, intelligence tests are descriptive, not explanatory. No intelligence test can indicate the reason for one's performance. To attribute inadequate performance on a test or in everyday-life activities to "inadequate intelligence" is a tautology. . . . (p. 6)

Tyler (1976) expresses her discontent in this statement:

Inimically, the more carefully we have standardized our testing procedures, the less likely we are to observe . . . alternative cognitive processes. . . . What I should like to see now is a loosening up of some of our rigid testing procedures. . . . To understand intelligence as a mental process and the ways individuals differ in their environments we must launch out in new directions, freeing ourselves from some of the psychometric fetters we have forged. (p. 25)

Dynamic assessment models represent one attempt to respond to this challenge. We are launched. Where we land and how well we fare are matters for future determination. We need to be clear in our goals, creative in our methods, and persistent in our values.

Part I of this text is now concluded. Parts II and III consist of manuals describing my models for dynamic assessment and for rating adult–child interactions. These are offered in experimental versions. Some research has been conducted with each, and these results are discussed where appropriate. Additional research is needed and welcome. Readers should be aware that the use of these approaches requires training and supervision.

II

MEDIATED LEARNING EXPERIENCE RATING SCALE MANUAL

INTRODUCTION

The Mediated Learning Experience (MLE) Rating Scale is my attempt to provide a means of assessing the degree to which MLE characterizes the interactions of any mediator with a young child. The concept of MLE derives from the theory of "structural cognitive modifiability" as described by Reuven Feuerstein and his colleagues (e.g., 1979, 1980). MLE is an attempt to account for the environmental and socialization experiences that have the potential to influence the cognitive development of children.

Feuerstein's definition from his 1979 text is as follows:

> Mediated learning experience . . . is defined as the interactional processes between the developing human organism and an experienced, intentioned adult who, by interposing himself between the child and external sources of stimulation, "mediates" the world to the child by framing, selecting, focusing, and feeding back environmental experiences in such a way as to produce in him appropriate learning sets and habits. (p. 71)

He amplifies this in his 1980 text as follows:

> . . . the way in which stimuli emitted by the environment are transformed by a "mediating" agent . . . [who], guided by his intentions, culture, and emotional investment, selects and organizes the world of stimuli for the child. The mediator selects stimuli that are most appropriate and then frames, filters, and schedules them. . . . Through this process . . . the cognitive structure of the child is affected. (pp. 15–16)

MLEs are contrasted with direct learning experiences, in which the child also engages. These types of experiences interact, in that optimal MLEs are predicted to enhance the child's ability to profit from direct experience. Cultural deprivation is defined in terms of the child's exposure to inadequate MLEs; no culture is inherently depriving, but distal circumstances such as poverty and illness may reduce an adult's ability to provide optimal MLEs, and thereby may negatively affect the child's cognitive development. However, it is the MLE that is interpreted as the direct or proximal influence on cognitive functioning, rather than associated factors such as organic states of the child or socioeconomic status (SES) of the family. These distal parameters affect the child's functioning through their effects on the delivery of or receptivity to MLEs.

Although Feuerstein's work has focused on late childhood through adolescence, and he is best known for demonstrating the cognitive modifiability of children and adults even at relatively late developmental stages, he has made the following statement that is relevant to the focus of the MLE Rating Scale on young children: "The more and earlier an organism is subjected to MLE, the greater will be his capacity to efficiently use and be affected by direct exposure to sources of stimuli" (1980, p. 16).

The MLE Rating Scale incorporates most of the components described by Feuerstein, but it reflects my own interpretations and modifications of this concept. Feuerstein never explicitly sought measurement of these factors, and the specifics he describes derive primarily from clinical experience and his expansions of a combination of theoretical influences (e.g., Piaget and Vygotsky). I have attempted to reconcile these clinical insights with research evidence (primarily from the parent–child interaction literature), as well as with a theory base derived from sources similar to Feuerstein's, but not conceptualized identically to his. The need for such a scale relates to several observations:

1. Most of the existing scales of adult–child interaction address interactions between mothers and infants. There is little that can be applied to children at older preschool ages and that is relevant to a broad array of mediators. The MLE Rating Scale has been used with mothers and teachers, and is about to be used with fathers and diagnostic assessors. It has been used in relation to children from the ages of 2 through 5, and has the potential for use with a broader age span.

2. Most of the existing scales include a narrow selection of interaction components. The MLE Rating Scale attempts to be a broad and comprehensive instrument—a summary of the multitude of factors occurring within teaching and parenting relationships that may influence the child's cognitive development.

3. Researchers and practitioners appear increasingly sensitive to the

need to join theory, assessment, intervention, and research. In the past, assessment tools were designed with little awareness of intervention issues and needs; interaction measures were limited to the research arena. Newly developing approaches in all areas of assessment try more systematically to link diagnosis with intervention, as well as to recognize the need to monitor progress and to evaluate intervention effectiveness. The MLE Rating Scale is designed to reflect all of these needs. It is usable as a diagnostic instrument to develop a profile of strengths and weaknesses of mediators. It is possible to move directly from diagnosis to intervention by using the components in a curriculum-referenced manner, as specific intervention objectives. Activities can be designed to enhance areas of need as indicated by the scale (see Appendix II.A for examples of home activities). It is then possible to use the scale to monitor progress and to evaluate intervention effectiveness.

4. Other scales rely either on complex coding systems, overly simple all-or-none checklists, or frequency counts. The MLE Rating Scale is intended to emphasize the qualitative nature of the mediator–child interaction, to be usable by practitioners in the field (i.e., without reliance on videotapes), to be easily taught and learned, and to yield meaningful information derived from brief observations. Therefore, a rating scale format has been selected. The highest rating within each category reflects the theoretically hypothesized optimal level of an MLE, and the highest ratings of all the components together reflect an operational definition of MLE.

An important deviation from Feuerstein's concepts and the scales of others who have attempted to evaluate MLEs is that this scale is designed only as a means of evaluating the mediator's contributions to the interaction. Although there is one global indicator of the child's contributions (reciprocity), the ratings on all other components are of the observed behaviors of the mediator. There is no intent to imply that influences on child development are unidirectional. It is well established that interactional effects are complex and multidirectional, and that children do not come into this world as blank slates. Therefore, other indicators are needed to reflect the child's contributions when the concerns are diagnostic or research-related, and there are times when more complex coding systems are relevant for capturing the complex interactional effects. What this scale is intended to provide is an evaluation of the mediator's behavioral repertory in areas thought to be relevant to the child's cognitive development. The assumption is that, despite the child's contributions, the adult mediator is likely to hold more power in the relationship, especially if the purpose of the observation is to devise an intervention program (Bell, 1979; Clarke-Stewart, 1973; Farran & Haskins, 1980). What the mediator does must always reflect the contribution of the child, and this in fact is built into the components of the scale; however, the focus of conscious change in the situation is on the mediator. Thus, there is no assumption of "cause" to be inferred (i.e., in terms of accounting for the characteristics of the initially observed interactions). The assumption is that, if change is desired, someone has to do something different, and the more reasonable target for effecting such change is the mediator.

Readers interested in a full consideration of approaches to assessment of MLE are referred to the work of other researchers investigating applications of MLE. These include Pnina S. Klein, at the School of Education, Bar Ilan University, Ramat Gan, Israel (Klein, no date; Klein & Feuerstein, 1985; Klein, Wieder, & Greenspan, 1987); Katherine Greenberg, at the University of Tennessee–Knoxville (Greenberg, 1987); Ruth Kahn, at St. Joseph College, West Hartford, Connecticut (Kahn, 1988); and Louis Falik, at San Francisco State University (Falik, 1989). David Tzuriel, at the School of Education, Bar Ilan University (Tzuriel & Eran, 1989), has also conducted research in this area, using Pnina Klein's scoring system. Additional elaboration on MLE by Feuerstein and his colleagues can be found in Feuerstein (1981), Feuerstein and Hoffman (1982), Feuerstein and Rand (1973–1975), and Feuerstein, Klein, and Tannenbaum (in press). A new journal that focuses on research into MLE and related issues is the *International Journal of Mediated Learning and Cognitive Education* (see the "Resources" section of this book for addresses from which to obtain this journal).

The MLE Rating Scale has been applied diagnostically in two different ways to date. Its first application has been as an observation tool in parent–child dyadic interactions. The parent (most often one parent, usually the mother, though sometimes both parents are observed) is asked to engage in two 10-minute interactions with the preschool child: spontaneous play with a standard set of age-appropriate toys, and a structured teaching interaction (e.g., building an animal from a model with bristle blocks or Legos; building a house with the same materials). The instructions for the play are as follows: "Please play with _____ as normally as you can, just as you would at home." The instructions for the teaching task are "Please teach _____ to make one just like this [picture on box]," or "Please teach _____ how to build a house with these blocks."

The length of time is fairly standard for observational research studies, and my impression is that the 10-minute span is sufficient to sample the repertory of most parents. Having two situations simply provides an opportunity for increased reliability and validity, as well as a chance to see the parent in two roles — as teacher and playmate. Some parents have difficulty differentiating the two, and this is diagnostically useful information. Parents are always debriefed after the observation, to give them an opportunity to inform the assessor of their perceptions of the validity of the experience, as well as to elaborate on any of the aspects of what occurred.

The second major diagnostic application of the MLE Rating Scale has been as a tool for observing teacher–child interactions, both in a one-to-one relationship and in large-group instruction. All of the components are relevant to both situations. Informal feedback from teachers has indicated that the scale is useful and meaningful. However, assessors must be careful to avoid use of the scale for "report card" evaluations of teachers. The intent of the scale is to generate feedback regarding a teacher's contribution to the instructional situation, and to generate recommendations regarding changes that may be helpful to facilitating the learning of the child, not to gather information reportable to the teacher's supervisor regarding her performance. Unless a teacher is glaringly neglectful or harmful, information derived from this approach should be held in confidence.

The third major application of the MLE Rating Scale has been for research. Three studies have been completed that included assessment of the psychometric properties of the scale, as well as research into interactional issues. Two more studies are planned — one to look at the usefulness of the scale for intervention planning and evaluation, and the second to investigate concurrent validity. These studies are described below. Readers are encouraged to conduct further investigations of the scale. Although it has evolved over several years of practice and study, it remains "experimental," and further work of course needs to be done.

A fourth potential application of the MLE Rating Scale is as a level-of-implementation indicator and training tool for dynamic assessment assessors. The intervention aspect of dynamic assessment, when used in its most clinical format and when derived from Feuerstein's model, is to provide an optimal MLE for the learner. When assessors are being trained to carry out dynamic assessment, and when research is being conducted in this area, the scale should be useful in providing a means of determining the extent to which an MLE is indeed taking place. It also provides an explicit definition for the assessor who is new to dynamic assessment of precisely what is meant by MLE (i.e., what it is that he is expected to be doing).

REVIEW OF RESEARCH
ON THE COMPONENTS OF MLE

Modifications of Feuerstein's Original Components

Although most of the components assessed by the MLE Rating Scale derive directly from the clinical work of Feuerstein and his colleagues, the literature provides much research evidence to justify the inclusion of the components on the scale. Some of this evidence has been reviewed elsewhere (Lidz, in press-a), but is included and further expanded upon below.

As noted earlier in this book (see Part I, Chapter 2), Feuerstein (1979, 1980; Jensen & Feuerstein, 1987) elaborates 10 components of MLE: mediation of intentionality and reciprocity; meaning; transcendence; feelings of competence; regulation of behavior; sharing; individuation and psychological differentiation; goal seeking, goal setting, and goal achievement; challenge; and change. (More recently, another component was added: mediation of a feeling of an optimistic alternative.) However, my reworking of the theoretical basis of dynamic assessment, the incorporation of MLE into the model as a guideline for assessor behavior, and research findings have all resulted in some modifications and reinterpretations of these components for the MLE Rating Scale. These include the following:

1. Goal setting, seeking, and achievement (and, by implication, planning) and regulation of behavior have been removed as separate components, and incorporated as the optimal states of *each* component. My reasoning was that goal-directedness, planning, and self-regulation are really the generally desired outcomes of the entire MLE process. The ultimate purpose of the mediated interaction is precisely to generate a self-regulating, active, strategic problem solver capable of representational thinking. Therefore, each component has been reinterpreted in terms of the extent to which these goals are promoted. Thus, the highest rating level within each component is the extent to which self-regulation and planning are facilitated. Rather than reducing the importance of these components by their removal, the MLE Rating Scale increases the importance of both by increasing their pervasiveness.

2. The component of mediation of competence has been expanded into three subcomponents, all having to do with enhancing the child's competence. At first, I intuitively decided that the subareas of praise/ encouragement and task regulation were separable; teachers and parents had been observed to be able to do one without necessarily involving the other. Subsequently, research demonstrated that these

did function separately and contributed differentially to the MLE profiles (Glazier-Robinson, 1986). I also decided that the idea of "challenge," so critical to Feuerstein's approach and to much of what is written in research on instruction, is really an aspect of mediation of competence; optimal challenge serves both as a motivation for change and as a source of direction for change, and the nature of the change is increased competence. Challenge is also easily interpreted in terms of Vygotsky's concept of "zone of proximal development" (ZPD; Minick, 1987) — one of the central theoretical bases underlying mediation and dynamic assessment, but not otherwise explicitly incorporated into the operationalization of the theory. Thus, there appear to be many faces of competence, each of which maintains some independence.

3. Reciprocity, although scored, is removed from calculation as an MLE component. First, the MLE Rating Scale, as indicated above, is conceived as a description of mediator behavior. Sensitivity to the child's contribution is built into the scale (e.g., contingent responsivity). It was also found in research (Glazier-Robinson, 1986) that reciprocity did not contribute to the scale's internal consistency to the extent that other components did. Although it is agreed that all the mediating behaviors in the world may be to no avail if the child is not receptive, it was felt that since the scale is merely a measure of the mediator's repertory, and sensitivity to the child is in fact represented, it is not necessarily the scale's mission to determine the degree of child responsiveness. The child's contribution needs to be noted and assessed in greater detail by alternative means; any conclusions or recommendations must take the child's responsiveness into consideration, but the intent of the scale is to describe mediator, not child, behavior.

4. I have been feeling confused regarding existing definitions of "transcendence" and "meaning," which often seem to overlap. In order to increase the clarity of interpretation and the scorability of these components, I decided (in consultation with Ruth Kahn) to make the determining issue the extent to which the concept or object of focus is perceivable within the situation. If the content of reference is perceivable, this is to be considered as "meaning"; if the referent requires conceptualization beyond the perceivable, this is "transcendence."

5. The component of sharing has also been expanded. One interpretation is an attempt to represent Feuerstein's idea as accurately as possible ("joint regard"). The second is my own alternative, more concrete interpretation ("shared experience"). Feuerstein's idea is more inferential, and it remains to be determined whether this can be reliably scored. My reinterpretation results in a behavior that occurs with very low frequency, and it remains to be determined whether this makes a meaningful contribution.

6. Finally, on the basis of a review of the research literature, two components have been added: affective involvement and contingent responsivity. The literature on parent–child interaction with young children provides consistently strong support for the contribution of these components to children's general competence and cognitive functioning (see below). I felt that a rating of characteristics purporting to represent the effective ingredients of influence could not ignore these very potent contributors.

Research Support for the Components *

Anyone who has looked at the literature on parent–child interaction has experienced the feeling of being overwhelmed by its sheer bulk, which increases daily. There is much substantiation within the literature of the relationship between parent–child interaction as generally conceived, and the cognitive, emotional, and social development of children (e.g., Clarke-Stewart, 1988; Bradley, Caldwell, & Rock, 1988). This review is limited to the specific characteristics of these interactions that seem to account for the relationship — specifically, the relationship of parent–child interaction to cognitive development. These specific characteristics are what define MLE, as represented by the MLE Rating Scale. This review is not comprehensive, but only representative of the available literature; the purpose is to provide evidence substantiating the inclusion of the specific components of the MLE Rating Scale.

Intentionality

When discussing the component of intentionality (usually paired with reciprocity), Feuerstein uses phrases such as "an experienced, intentioned adult who . . . [interposes] himself between the child and external sources of stimulation" (1979, p. 71). Klein and Feuerstein (1985) use the phrase "the intention to mediate," elaborating that "MLE is clearly not accidental; it is a conscious intentioned act. It is a dynamic process in which the mediator . . . attempts a series of actions to reach the objective of . . . mediation" (p. 372). With these statements in mind, intentionality is interpreted here to indicate the adult's active attempts to influence the child, and behaviors involved in maintaining the child's involvement in the interaction. Thus, behaviors involved in initiating, maintaining, and terminating the interaction, as well as in

*Portions of this section appear in Lidz (in press-a).

regulating and refocusing the child's attention and participation, are included in this component.

Research literature that relates to this component includes the following. DeLoache and DeMendoza (1987), in their study of 30 mother–child dyads (with children aged 12, 15, and 18 months) involved in a picture book task, found that in all three groups the mothers controlled and took primary responsibility for the interaction. Heckhausen's (1987) study, which also related to contingent responsivity, showed how mothers adjusted the level of their involvement to the level of perceived competence of the children, providing more supports when the children showed difficulty, and fading out involvement when the children demonstrated mastery. Kuczynski (1984) found that mothers' use of reasoning as a control strategy was associated with the imposition of long-term versus short-term goals, and that the children who experienced reasoning were more compliant, were less negative, and used negotiation as a strategy for themselves. This study involved 64 dyads with college graduate mothers and their 4-year-old children. The reasoning components that were most effective included providing a rationale for the activity and referring to social values or intrinsic worth of the task. This supports the value of a more distal, rule-related strategy as opposed to a directly physical strategy for induction of self-regulation in the child. Similar results were obtained by Kuczynski, Kochanska, Radke-Yarrow, and Girnius-Brown (1987) in a study of 70 mother–child dyads with a younger population (children aged $1\frac{1}{2}$ to $3\frac{1}{2}$ years). Again, direct control strategies were associated with defiance as a means of resistance, whereas reasoning was associated with negotiation. Levenstein's (1979) results demonstrated that the mother descriptor "tries to converse with child" was one of the three most important contributors to a child's task and cognitive orientation.

Maccoby, Snow, and Jacklin (1984) observed 57 mother–infant dyads in a teaching task when the children were 12 and 18 months of age. They recorded the nature of the teaching provided, which included demonstrating, providing physical help, making requests, imposing demands, and "directing." These researchers found no relationship between the "total teaching effort" variable (which summarized positive, negative, and direct teaching) at 12 months and task orientation at 18 months (i.e., this variable was not predictive), but did find a significant concurrent relationship between total teaching effort at 18 months and the child's task orientation at 18 months. They noted that the parents' behavior at 12 months was better characterized by caretaking than by teaching. However, those mothers who did engage in a high teaching effort at the younger age had children who were temperamentally less difficult at the older age. Rocissano and Yatchmink (1983) reported a relationship between mothers' ability to sustain joint focus with their 24-month-old prematurely born children, and the children's language development. And, finally, Slade (1987) demonstrated that in 16 mother–child dyads engaged in 30-minute play sessions (the children were seen bimonthly between the ages of 20 and 28 months), a mother's presence and involvement (via active interaction or verbal commentary) was associated with an increase in the length and level of a child's play.

Although none of these studies specifically used the term "intentionality," they do provide evidence that the mothers' effort to teach and control the interaction was associated with increased task involvement of the children. Furthermore, the nature of the mothers' control strategies — that is, reasoning versus physical control — related positively to the children's development of self-regulation.

Meaning

Feuerstein (1980) wrote the following about mediation of meaning: "Certain stimuli are selected by the mother as being more relevant and meaningful than others . . . and, therefore, a background is provided against which categorization becomes possible at later stages of development" (p. 27). Jensen and Feuerstein (1987) pointed out that mediation of meaning relates to the energetic, motivational aspects of the interaction, explained by Klein and Feuerstein (1985) as follows:

> The objects that surround a child have *no* meaning to him or her unless they bear meaning to the mediator. . . . A child has to learn to expect relations between what is perceived or experienced and affective connotations and undertones that may derive from cultural values or other parental experiences. (p. 373)

Through mediation of meaning, the child learns the attributed cultural values of what is good and bad, what is important to note, and what can be ignored; important cognitive outcomes of mediation of meaning include the ability to compare and to categorize, based on perceptions and explanations of how events and objects relate.

Literature relating to the component of meaning includes a study by Carew (1980), who found a significant relationship between the parenting behaviors of "labeling objects and relationships" (p. 68) and children's intellectual development at 3 years. Hess and Shipman (1968) wrote:

> The cognitive environment of the culturally disadvantaged child is one in which behavior is controlled by imperatives rather than [by] the

individual characteristics of a specific situation, and one in which behavior is neither mediated by verbal cues . . . nor mediated by teaching that relates events to one another and the present to the future. The meaning of deprivation would thus seem to be a deprivation of meaning. . . . (p. 102)

In a later study, Hess and Shipman (1973) found that their middle-class parents differed from their lower-SES parents in the latter's failure to relate one act to another; they concluded that "in this sense it [the interaction] lacks meaning; it is not sufficiently related to the context in which it occurs, to the motivations of the participants, or to the goals of the task" (p. 36).

Although the definition of "meaning" provided by the MLE Rating Scale differs somewhat from these authors' interpretations of the term, the aspect of attribution of importance and value is inherent, as well as the communication of this through affect and explanation. When mediators communicate to children what is important to notice, with additional elaboration of descriptive characteristics and related information to promote understanding, the adults have mediated meaning. This becomes transcendence when the information requires conceptualization of elements not present in the situation, or involves cause-and-effect or inferential thinking.

Transcendence

In Feuerstein's early writing (1979), he linked transcendence with intentionality, describing MLE primarily in terms of the "intent to transcend" the current situation and the child's immediate needs. Somewhat later, Feuerstein (1980) wrote that "there is nothing in our biological existence that necessitates abstract thinking. . . . Such processes arise in response to cultural needs. . . . Therefore, MLE is directly responsible for the functioning that transcends the biological needs of the individual" (p. 26). He added that transcendence may involve communication of the concepts of time (now vs. later) and space (here vs. there) (1980, p. 26). Transcendence may also involve communication regarding past events either within or beyond the child's own experiences, as well as encouragement of projection into the future. This allows the child not only to conceptualize events that cannot be seen, but to relate events in the current situation to those in the past or anticipated in the future; both of these abilities are antithetical to the cognitive dysfunction of "episodic grasp of reality," observed to be characteristic of poor learners.

Sigel and his colleagues have developed their concept of "distancing

strategies" parallel to and quite similar to Feuerstein's conceptualization
of "transcendence." In fact, in one publication, Sigel even uses the term
"transcendence." In 1979, McGillicuddy-DeLisi, Sigel, and Johnson
defined "distancing" to

> include those classes of behavior that "demand" the child to reconstruct
> past events, to employ his imagination in dealing with objects, events,
> and people, to plan and anticipate future actions . . . and, finally, to
> attend to the transformation of phenomena. Distancing behaviors make
> a demand on the child to infer from the observable present, and, in the
> course of making such inferences, the child has to present to himself the
> outcomes or reconstructions of previous events. (p. 98)

Sigel and McGillicuddy-DeLisi (1984) have applied this definition to
specific parenting behaviors as follows:

> Parental verbalizations that focus on getting the child to pose alterna-
> tives, to evaluate consequences, to infer cause–effect, to plan, etc. . . .
> are higher level distancing strategies for a preschool child because they
> encourage greater psychological distance from the present concrete
> situation, as well as demand greater representational ability. . . . (p. 76)

And, in 1986, Sigel defines representation as

> internalization of experience and subsequent competence in three func-
> tions: anticipation, hindsight, and transcendance [sic] of the ongoing
> present . . . [that includes] the understanding of the rule that experience
> can be transformed into various sign and symbol systems and that
> instances retain a core identity in spite of the transformation. (pp.
> 51–52)

Sigel and his colleagues have produced an impressive array of
research data to document the association between parental distancing
strategies and the cognitive development of preschool children. Some of
their findings include the following: a relationship between the use of
distancing strategies and family size (single-child families did more
than families with three children); greater use by mothers than by
fathers; variations in use related to the amount of structure of the task
(more distancing with less structure); and a positive relationship
between the use of distancing strategies and the child's competence on
a series of problem-solving tasks (McGillicuddy-DeLisi et al., 1979).
Sigel and McGillicuddy-DeLisi (1984), in summarizing the results of
three projects involving 360 families with 4-year-old children, noted
higher occurrence of distancing with a paper-folding than with a

storytelling task; higher occurrence of distancing between parents and their cross-gender children; adjusted reduction of distancing strategies with communication-handicapped children; and a significant relationship between use of distancing strategies and Wechsler Preschool and Primary Scale of Intelligence (WPPSI) IQs (strongest for the communication-handicapped group).

Although Sigel and colleagues provide the bulk of information relating to transcendence, Ratner (1980) also reports related findings in results showing an association between parental references to past events and use of the word "remember," and their children's memory development.

Competence

According to Jensen and Feuerstein (1987),

> By ensuring conditions for successful interaction, [the mediator] creates a climate wherein a feeling of competency follows successful mastery. In order to enlist impulses of mastery and a motive to achieve, [the mediator] . . . organizes opportunities for success, and through the mediation of competence following mastery, produces within the individual the expectancies of success which will enhance the learner's ability to effect transfer. (p. 387)

Along with the outcome of feelings of mastery comes increased willingness to explore and to attack challenge (Klein & Feuerstein, 1985). The mediator not only informs the child regarding correctness or evaluates the child's efforts, but focuses "on the processes that led to success and on the mental process that preceded it" (Klein & Feuerstein, 1985, p. 374).

Feuerstein and his colleagues discuss two aspects of mediation of feelings of competence. First, the mediator manipulates the task or situation to increase the child's probability of mastery. This has been incorporated into the MLE Rating Scale as "task regulation." Second, the mediator offers encouragement and praise, which have been incorporated into the scale using these same terms. Within each of these areas, optimal mediation provides information regarding the processes and behaviors that have led to these successes or failures, in order to promote self-regulation and transfer of learning to new situations.

Finally, as noted earlier, I have incorporated Feuerstein's component of "challenge" under the general heading of mediation of competence. This is not a deviation from Feuerstein's conceptualization, since he and Jensen discuss this component as "drawing upon the mediation of competence" (Jensen & Feuerstein, 1987, p. 388). Challenge is seen in terms of encouraging the child's "propensity to seek out tasks for their novelty and complexity . . . above and beyond the mediation of competence to overcome the insecurity and anxiety associated with the unfamiliar" (Jensen & Feuerstein, 1987, p. 388). I have expanded this conceptualization of challenge to include the notions of "scaffolding" (e.g., Wood, 1980; Wood, Bruner, & Ross, 1976) and the "ZPD" (e.g., Minick, 1987; Wertsch, 1979).

The concept of scaffolding describes the mediator's adjusting the complexity and difficulty of the teaching interaction to facilitate the child's mastery of the task; providing support when necessary; and providing encouragement and prompts to the child to move ahead when ready. The notion of ZPD, discussed briefly in Chapter 1 of Part I, describes the mediator's maintenance of interaction within the child's ability to respond with adult help. The mediator reduces interaction when the child is able to function independently, and increases interaction to facilitate the child's ability to move ahead and beyond her current level. The ZPD describes the parameters within which the mediator may productively function, as well as the range of the child's ability to respond with and without mediator intervention. The mediator's manipulation of the task and of the teaching parameters is described by the competency component of task regulation. The maintenance of these maneuvers within the child's ZPD is described by the component of challenge, and the correct reading of the child's needs and timely response to these needs is described by the component of contingent responsivity, to be discussed below. It is thus possible for a mediator to make a number of task manipulations (thus scoring high on this component), and to make these moves in timely response to the child's needs (thus scoring high on contingent responsivity), but to place these maneuvers above or below the child's ZPD (therefore scoring low on challenge).

Research that relates to competence as task regulation includes a study by Heckhausen (1987), who showed that provision of supports by parents to balance weaknesses fostered very young children's development; with increasing age of his subjects (within their second year), the parental aids became more verbal and less physical.

Literature relating to competence as praise and encouragement includes a study by Feshbach (1973), who found a significant relationship between mothers' and children's use of negative statements in the teaching situation; he also found that mothers of poor readers made more negative statements even when teaching children of other parents. Finkelstein and Ramey (1977) found that immediate positive feedback enhanced infant learning abilities. Norman-Jackson (1982) found that parents of children who developed into successful readers made fewer discouragements of their children's verbalizations. Olson, Bates, and Bayles (1984) reported that parents who were relatively nonpunitive had the most competent toddlers. Ramey, Farran, and Campbell (1979) demonstrated that absence of punishment was the most significant contributor at 6 months in their day care group and at 18 to 20 months in their home care group to prediction of Stanford–Binet IQ at 36 months. Streissguth and Bee (1971) related maternal patterns of positive feedback and the parents' use of questions to the children's cognitive performance. Hitz and Driscoll (1988) discuss the many controversial aspects of use of praise, and suggest that "effective praise" provides information and descriptive feedback to the child; it also includes relatively few evaluative comments that induce reliance on external judgments.

Research relating to mediation of competence as challenge includes the work of Heckhausen (1987), who investigated the mother–child teaching interaction as an apprenticeship model within the framework of Vygotsky's ZPD. He specifically focused on the characteristics of provision of support and provision of challenge in a study of mothers with their 2-year-old children. Challenge was defined in terms of a "one-step-ahead strategy," with a focus of instruction "on those aspects of the task that were just beyond the level of mastery currently attained by their infants" (p. 763). In this longitudinal study, taking place over an 8-month period, Heckhausen's mothers followed the one-step-ahead strategy: Instructions became increasingly cognitively demanding as the children's mastery increased, and the challenge strategy required higher levels of inference by the children. Heckhausen concluded that "in the present study the mothers' objective was not just to maximize the number of children's successes by balancing for their weaknesses but, additionally, to sustain a level of challenge that they deemed to be most promotive of the child[ren]'s development across the changes in their competence" (1987, p. 770). The work of Sigel and colleagues cited above also supports the notion of challenge as related to the child's cognitive development, and several citations in Clarke-Stewart (1973) support the relationship between cognitive development and parental teaching strategies that are cognitively demanding.

Sharing

Sharing, interpreted as "joint regard" and "sharing experiences" on the MLE Rating Scale, is described by Jensen and Feuerstein (1987) as

> the energetic component, that, through examiner–examinee eye contact, pointing, and tracking, enables the mediator to impart stimuli selected

by intent. . . . The mediation of sharing in the . . . interaction contributes to the establishment within the [child] of need systems to communicate with others and the propensity to search for the appropriate tempo
and modality to overcome egocentricity. (pp. 387–388)

Feuerstein (1987) further elaborates sharing as the mediator's sharing
of views, feelings, reactions, and gaze—focus on the same object.
Sharing includes synchronization of movements, encouragement of
sharing of feelings and perceptions from the child, and demonstrations
of how to do this for the child. Sharing begins with joint regard,
sharing of experiences, and communication to the child that the
interaction is a jointly shared experience.

Because sharing is such a complex and multifaceted component, I
decided to divide it into the dual aspects of "joint regard" and "sharing
of experiences," to represent more clearly the varieties of the types of
sharing that are possible. Research support for this component includes
the study by Carew (1980), who specifically mentions that sharing of
information by mothers was one of the parenting behaviors most
closely associated with children's intellectual development. Also, Friedman, Gordon, and Ross (1986) have specified initiation and maintenance of "shared focus" as a central component of maternal teaching,
and have defined this variable as follows: (1) The mother and child
indicate via observable behavior (including speech) that they are
attending to each other, and (2) both mother and child are attending to
some common object or event and are aware of each other's attending
to the same event. These researchers present data based on 8-minute
observations of interactions in mother–child dyads, and conclude that

> most of the time was spent in shared focus and the episodes of shared
> attention lasted for an average of 84.6 seconds. It is quite apparent . . .
> that mothers have an important role as collaborators in initiating,
> maintaining, and terminating a shared focus. They do not, however,
> have a leading role. (p. 5)

Also relating to the component of sharing, Stern (1984), using his
term "affect attunement," described his exploratory observational study
of 10 mother–child dyads: When questioned about their behavior, the
mothers said that they were trying to join, participate, and "be with"
their infants. He demonstrated the importance of a good sharing match
in deliberately inducing a mismatch of mothers' attunement and
observing the children's awareness when this occurred. Stern views
attunement as relating to the infant's development of a capacity for
intimacy and a sense of self.

Finally, Tomasello and Farrar (1986) reported a relationship between maternal references to objects within the children's focus and the vocabulary development of the children. These children were between the ages of 15 and 21 months.

Psychological Differentiation

Feuerstein, Rand, and Rynders (1988) describe the component of individuation and psychological differentiation as "in some respects, the opposite of sharing. Sharing is fusion between two people; individuation and differentiation put the emphasis on how we distinguish ourselves from others" (p. 78). Jensen and Feuerstein (1987) refer to differentiation in terms of mediating "the child's capacity for and right to a dualistic organism–world relationship" (p. 388). These descriptions have been interpreted for inclusion in the MLE Rating Scale in terms of the degree to which the mediator encourages and enables the child to function as an independent entity rather than as an extension of the mediator, and, along with this, the ability of the mediator to maintain an objective stance in the interaction. This requires a lack of intrusiveness on the part of the mediator, as well as acceptance — even encouragement — of differences and alternative points of view. The concept was beautifully, even poetically, phrased by a $4\frac{1}{2}$-year-old girl (quoted by Feuerstein et al., 1988) when she expressed her anger to her grandmother with her failure to learn to peel a potato:

> "I am not you
> and you are not me.
> Your hand is not mine
> and my hand is not yours.
> And you can't do things like me
> and I can't do things like you
> and that's it." (p. 78)

And that pretty much says "it," in the words of a well-differentiated child.

Research literature that relates to the component of differentiation includes the work of Bayley and Schaefer (1964), who cited a negative relationship for girls between maternal intrusiveness and IQ, and of Streissguth and Bee (1971), who concluded that the extent to which the mother became physically involved with the task "seems to have strong implications for the child's feeling of participation and autonomy" (p. 159). Also, Wood (1980) found that one of three components of successful maternal teaching was the "*progressive relaxation of adult control over . . . problem solving,"* which gave "the child a sense of competence by offering him initiative, giving him options to choose between, and providing him with a framework for interpreting his experience" (p. 295; italics in original).

Change

The component of change (or mediation of an awareness of the human being as a changing entity) relates to the feedback aspect of the mediation of competence; however, this component specifically involves feedback related to the child's ability to learn and to become modified by the teaching interaction. Mediation of change allows the child to leave the situation with the feeling of being able to learn and to profit from experience. To accomplish this requires

> constant and fine grained feedback regarding performance. . . . Failure is acknowledged but limited in its input to the specific behaviors or deficient functions which produced it. Successes are amplified and attributed to the . . . child's growing mastery. The mediation of change is undertaken to equip the child with insight into his/her growing proficiency. (Jensen & Feuerstein, 1987, p. 389)

No literature specific to this component has been located. The component of change therefore remains hypothetical in terms of its relationship to cognitive development; however, it has strong intuitive appeal, and is recommended for more focused attention in future research.

Regulation of Behavior and Goal Seeking, Setting, and Achievement

Mediation of the regulation of behavior, and mediation of goal seeking, setting, and achievement, are described as components of MLE by Feuerstein and his colleagues. However, as indicated above, I have decided that, since these actually represent the outcomes of the entire mediational process, they should be built into each of the components of the MLE Rating Scale rather than being considered separately.

Mediation of behavior regulation concerns efforts to gain and maintain the child's attention and involvement in the task and to inhibit impulsive behavior, and, ultimately, to do so in a way that develops self-regulation within the child. The aspects of attention regulation and impulse regulation are viewed as inseparable from the component of intentionality, and are therefore described above as related to this component. The literature supportive of the relevance of self-regulation, as an outcome of this as well as other components, includes a study by Camp, Swift, and Swift (1982), who found a significant negative association between mothers' authoritarian attitudes and their children's IQs. These authors defined authoritarian attitude in terms of an emphasis on external control, with little verbal reasoning. Also, Levenstein (1979) found the maternal descriptor "verbalizes reasons for obedience" to be one among the three most important contributors to children's task and cognitive orientation.

The relevance of planning, subsuming the variable of goal orientation, to cognitive development and definition is elaborated in detail in Part III of this book. Hess and Shipman (1973) found that their low-SES mothers differed significantly from their middle-class mothers regarding the taking of time for reflection and planning. The cognitive literature during the last several years has provided strong support for the association of the ability to reflect, plan, and strategize with successful learning (Lidz, 1987b).

Contingent Responsivity

The concept of "contingent responsivity" refers to the ability of the mediator to respond to the child's behavior in both a timely and an appropriate way. The research literature on parent–child interaction, particularly in reference to infants and young children, is replete with discussion and support for this variable and its relationship with cognitive development.

Lewis (1978) specifies four dimensions of contingent responsivity: consistency, latency, relation to occurrence, and nature. "Consistency" refers to the "repeated pairing of specific action with specific outcomes" (p. 470). With regard to latency, Lewis points out the possibility that responses that are too slow may go beyond the infant's memory span of about 5 seconds, whereas responses that are too fast may occur within the recovery period and may thus interfere with processing. With regard to nature and outcome, Lewis assumes that some outcomes are inherently better than others in terms of the "prewiring" of the organism (e.g., receipt of food in response to vocalization signaling hunger; pp. 476–477). Lewis provides data documenting the positive relationship between maternal interactive behaviors that include responsivity and infant Bayley Mental Development Index scores, derived from in-home observations over a 2-hour span of time.

There is a great deal of literature dealing with this component. Bakeman and Brown (1980) found an association between mothers' emotional and verbal responsiveness when the children were 20 months of age, and both social and cognitive development of the children at 3 years. Bornstein and Tamis-LeMonda (1989) found a positive relationship between maternal responsivity and speed of habituation of the infants, as well as novelty preference of the infants. Furthermore, these researchers found that maternal responsiveness in infancy predicted toddler representational competence above and beyond other forms of stimulation. Interestingly, and related to the content of this material, Bornstein and Tamis-LeMonda also reported a stronger relationship between responsiveness and a learning measure than between responsiveness and WPPSI IQ, although both were strongly positive. Bradley and Caldwell (1976) reported that the aspects of the home environment that related most strongly to IQ were emotional and verbal responsivity of the mother, maternal involvement with the child, and provision of appropriate play materials. In a more recent article, Bradley (1989) discusses caretaker responsiveness as moderately stable across a number of years, and related to children's cognitive development between the ages of 2 and $4\frac{1}{2}$. Clarke-Stewart (1973) reported findings of a high degree of relationship between a mother's contingent responsivity and a child's competence.

Further evidence comes from the following studies. Gottfried (1985) conducted a meta-analysis of studies relating home environment to cognitive development and found play materials, maternal involvement, and maternal responsivity to be the three most significant variables. Levenstein (1979) found the maternal descriptor "responds to child's requests" to be one of the three most important contributors to children's task and cognitive orientation in her study. Lewis and Goldberg (1969) reported significant positive associations between the responsiveness of a mother to her infant's crying and vocalization and the infant's cognitive development; there was also a positive association between the rapidity of the response and cognitive development. Olson et al. (1984) found that maternal verbal and emotional responsivity when children were 6 months of age was significantly correlated with the children's cognitive competence at 2 years. Pratt, Kerig, Cowan, and Cowan (1988) showed not only that the parents they studied maintained their interactions within the children's ZPD, but documented the relationship between the parents' ability to adapt their interventions to the children's successes and failures and the children's overall success on the tasks.

Vietze and Anderson (1981) cited much evidence to support the relationship between a mother's responsivity and a child's cognitive functioning, and specified 10 seconds from the onset of the child's behavior as a definition of "contingent." Yarrow, Morgan, Jennings, Harmon, and Gaiter (1982) found associations between maternal and object responsiveness and stimulation at 6 months on the one hand, and infant task persistence and competence at 13 months on the other. And, finally, Yarrow, Rubenstein, Pederson, and Jankowski (1972) reported significant positive relationships among mental development, level and variety of social stimulation, and contingent response to distress. Contingent response to distress also related to goal-directed behavior, but not to exploratory behavior. However, contingent response to positive vocalization was related to exploratory behavior.

Thus, if we are seeking to identify and represent the most potent contributors to cognitive development in the infant and young child's interpersonal environment, contingent responsivity of the primary caretakers is certainly a strong candidate.

Affective Involvement

There is yet another candidate for inclusion on the list of potent contributors to cognitive development that has received strong research support: affective involvement. This is describable as the "warmth" factor, and differs from the affective contribution to the component of meaning. In the case of meaning, affect is involved to provide emphasis and notation of importance. In the case of affective involvement, the mediator communicates a sense of caring and emotional involvement with the child; this need not be extroverted, but should be perceptible in the look, gesture, and/or verbalizations of the mediator. The assumption is that a child will learn more from a mediator who seems to care for him than from one who is indifferent or hostile.

Research support for inclusion of this component comes from three main sources: evidence of explicit relationships; inferences from research involving maternal depression; and research focusing on attachment.

Research involving direct relationships includes the work of Bayley and Schaefer (1964), who showed a positive relationship in their longitudinal data between evidence of affection and a loving relationship during infancy and late preschool IQ for boys; in the case of girls, there was only such evidence concurrently during infancy. Lewis and Fox (1980) cited a number of studies that "attempt to establish a relationship between the emotional tone that pervades maternal behavior and infant intellectual development. Most of these studies have related ratings of 'positive emotional effect,' 'warmth,' or 'degree of involvement' with intellectual development" (p. 57). Stern, Caldwell, Hersher, Lipton, and Richmond (1969) conducted a factor-analytic study of mothers and their 1-year-old infants, looking at 79 variables for 30 mother–child dyads. They found that nine factors accounted for

64.6% of the variance; one of the primary factors was "lovingness," which included affective involvement as a component.

Research involving maternal depression includes that of Cox, Puckering, Pound, and Mills (1987), who found that depressed mothers were less responsive and less able to sustain social interaction than nondepressed mothers; their children were more often distressed and showed delays in expressive language development, as well as more emotional and behavioral disturbance. Rutter (1990) summarizes research reported in a special journal issue on maternal depression as follows: "Depressed mothers tend to be less positive with their new babies. . . . depressed mother–infant dyads spend more time together in negative affective states. . . . parenting qualities were associated with variations in children's social behavior" (p. 60). Later in the article, Rutter elaborates on possible reasons for these findings:

> Depression is associated with impairments in parenting through several different mechanisms. . . . First, the negative mood experienced by the mothers may lead directly to a negative shift in the affect expressed toward their infants. . . . Second, the depressive mood may diminish mothers' sensitivity and responsivity to children's cues and needs . . . , impair their disciplinary functioning . . . , or lead them inappropriately to use their infants as sources of comfort. . . . Third, because depression is associated with family discord . . . , the associated increase in conflict may impinge adversely on the offspring. . . . Fourth, there may be parenting difficulties that stem from the social adversities or the impairments in social functioning that create the increased risk for depression. . . . (pp. 61–62)

And, finally, in a study of parents with a history of psychiatric disorder (not necessarily depression), Baldwin, Cole, and Baldwin (1982) found that a significant predictor of the child's school functioning was the "warmth" factor. They concluded that "active/warm parent–child interaction, especially active/warm father–child interaction, is related to the children's school adjustment, particularly the ratings of cognitive function and motivation" (p. 79).

The third source of information regarding the relationship between affective involvement and the child's cognitive development comes from the literature on attachment. For example, Clarke-Stewart (1973) reported a positive relationship between positive affect expressed toward a child at 11 months and variables such as cognitive performance, secure attachment, and expression of positive affect at 12 months. Zaslow, Rabinovich, Suwalsky, and Klein (1988) observed parents with their 12-month-old first-born infants in their homes and found that mothers of insecure/avoidant children had more negative affective expression during the observation and were less playful with their infants. The presence of fathers was associated with fewer shows of negative affect. Finally, long-term effects of warmth on academic functioning have been reported by Estrada, Arsenio, Hess, and Holloway (1987) and Maccoby and Martin (1983).

Concluding Comments

In closing this review, I should note that it is not only what parents do that is important to a child's development; an assessor must also be aware of the beliefs and knowledge base from which these behaviors derive. Although the overt behaviors may provide information about the controlling variables in child development, it may not be sufficient to note behaviors without consideration of the cognitive basis for these actions when there is an intent to link diagnosis with intervention. It is unlikely that intervention can be effective without addressing these additional factors (Goldberg, 1982; Miller, 1988). For example, Goldberg (1982) reported the results of a study showing that parents' beliefs about their role as educators of their children were related to the preparedness of their children for school. Specifically, parents who believed that it was their job to teach specific content had children who not only scored higher on tests of this content, but were also rated higher by their teachers on general verbal skills. Thus, although the MLE Rating Scale may be useful in outlining the observable behaviors of parents interacting with young children, it needs to be supplemented with additional measures when used in relation to an intervention program. Sources for information on parents' knowledge about child development, and beliefs about their roles as parents and about children, include the following: Epstein (1980); Hess, Kashiwagi, Azuma, Price, and Dickson (1980); Johnson and Martin (1985); MacPhee (1981); and McGillicuddy-DeLisi (1985).

GUIDELINES FOR SCORING MLE COMPONENTS

I have tried to be as explicit as possible in designing the MLE Rating Scale, to enable raters to evaluate mediator–child interactions from direct reference to the scale. However, it is inevitable that questions arise and that further clarifications are needed. What follows is additional elaboration and discussion to help clarify the scoring of the MLE components, based on experience with training raters and using the scale in practice. It is impossible to anticipate all the possible circumstances that will arise in attempting to apply this scale. The intent here is to provide guidelines to facilitate raters' decision making in a broad variety of circumstances.

Intentionality

Intentionality is one of the more easily scored of the components. However, raters need to be careful that they do not assign the highest rating unless the mediator states a general principle that can potentially be internalized by the child to develop self-regulation. Statements such as "Let's move this closer so you can reach all the pieces by yourself," or "Why don't we try putting out just the pieces you need, so you aren't tempted to touch everything?" or "I notice that you work much better when you stand up every once in a while," would qualify for the highest rating. These qualify because the child can eventually tell herself to stand up, or move the pieces closer, or move herself closer, without reliance on external reminders. The essence of intentionality is the effort to keep the interaction going and to keep the child involved; this necessarily involves maintaining the child's attention, inhibiting impulsive behavior, and maintaining a goal orientation. Raters are reminded that a mediator should not be assigned a low rating when the child is already self-regulated; in this case, the parent who shows a readiness to become involved as needed should be assigned a score of 2, and, if any principle reinforcing self-regulation is offered, then a score of 3 is warranted.

Meaning

An important factor to keep in mind when scoring meaning is that the references need to apply to what can be perceived in the situation; it is often the case that statements are simultaneously scorable for both meaning and transcendence when they include both references to the perceivable and references to the imaginable. Statements such as "Oh, this is really funny!" or elaborations such as "Look how thick these crayons are; that makes them easier for you to hold," would qualify in the former case for a 2, and, in the latter for a 3. Moving an object around and attributing sound effects, such as barking sounds after the building of a dog is completed, would warrant a 2. When labels are provided, these should be references to what the child already knows in order to be scorable as "meaning." This may not always be readily determined; when the rater is in doubt, the mediator should be granted the score. Provision of additional information about the object or picture could qualify as meaning or transcendence, depending upon the demands on perception or conception.

Transcendence

Transcendence appears to be one of the most sensitive components to SES differences; it seems to occur with low frequency among lower-SES parents, and with very high frequency within the higher-SES populations. The most important factor in scoring transcendence is that there are cognitive demands on conceptualization that take the child beyond the currently perceivable situation. If the mediator simply says, "Oh, remember when we did that last week?" that is scored as a 1. If the mediator elaborates with "When we went to the park last week, you made sure you tried all of the games, but you had the most fun on the swings. Remember?" that would rate a 2. If the mediator says something like "Remember when we went to the playground last week and we only had two trikes for the whole class? What did we have to do?", that would rate a 3 because the elaborated reference requires additional inferential and cause-and-effect thinking on the part of the child.

Sharing (Joint Regard)

Simple attempts to "join" the child are scored either 1 or 2, depending upon the presence of elaboration. In order to obtain a 3, the mediator needs to express an empathic inference — for example, "Wow, you were afraid you couldn't do that, but you tried anyway," or "I know you're saying you're tired, but I really think you feel this is too hard."

Sharing (Shared Experience)

The component of shared experience involves a statement by the mediator of a thought or experience of the mediator's. A statement such as "I used to play with something like this when I was your age" would qualify for a 1. If there is elaboration, such as "The blocks that we used to have when I was little were much stronger than these; they didn't fall apart so quickly," this would qualify for a 2. A statement such as "I used to think that dolls were just for girls, and that if I played with them I would turn into a girl! Isn't that silly!" would qualify for a 3. Remarks do not necessarily need to refer to the past in order to be scored for this component. If the mediator shares a contemporary thought, this is scorable as well.

Competence (Task Regulation)

The important thing to keep in mind when scoring task regulation is that the mediator must either state a principle of problem solution or induce strategic thinking in the child in order to be scored at the highest level. This does not require an elaborate statement. A remark such as "Where shall we start? What should be do first?" would qualify. Statement of a principle, such as "This will be more stable if we start from the bottom," or "You need to press down really hard on the blocks so they will hold together" in relation to Legos or bristle blocks, would qualify for a 3. These latter qualify because they provide a rule that is potentially internalizable by the child to facilitate self-regulation and transfer to other similar tasks.

Competence (Praise/Encouragement)

The difference between a 2 and a 3 in the component of praise/encouragement is again the statement of a general principle. In the case of a 3, frequency is not as important as the provision of a general rule. Therefore, many exclamations of "Great!" or "Good job!" would warrant a 2, whereas one statement such as "You really slowed down and worked carefully; great job!" would warrant a 3.

Competence (Challenge)

The component of challenge is included in the scale only when it is used for teachers and assessors, because the length of observation time in the case of parent–child dyads is not considered sufficient to elicit this component. Also, the nature of the activities engaged in by parent–child dyads is not always conducive to elicitation of this component. Challenge is sometimes difficult to distinguish from task regulation and contingent responsivity. Task regulation refers to the actual directions and intervention provided by the mediator, whether within the child's optimal ZPD range or not; it is possible to obtain a high score on task regulation, but a low score on challenge. Contingent responsivity refers to the flexibility of the mediator—that is, the adjustment of the mediator's behavior in response to the cues emitted by the child. These moves may indicate an appropriate reading of the child's signals, yet may not provide an instructional challenge. Thus, the component of challenge refers to the optimal match between the presentation of the task and the child's ability to respond, balancing support with challenge, providing a "one-step-ahead" kind of strategy.

Psychological Differentiation

The component of psychological differentiation refers to the "intrusiveness" of the mediator; this is usually more of an issue for parents than for teachers or examiners. However, a low rating on this component would be appropriate for teachers as well, in a case when the product becomes more important than the process. Parents who take on the task as theirs and forget that their role is to facilitate a learning experience for the child have difficulty with this component. A few parents have even been observed to reject the efforts of their children to become involved, and in this case, a minus score has been introduced.

Contingent Responsivity

Contingent responsivity is one of the most inferential of the components. This component refers to the "dance" between a child who behaves and a mediator who reads the child's behavior and reacts in a timely and appropriate way. Mediators are not expected to react to every single instance of child behavior; however, there should be an overall impression of a mediator who is tuned in to and responsive to the child, so that the child is left with a feeling of being able to influence and eventually to predict the effects.

Affective Involvement

The component of affective involvement, as noted earlier, reflects the "warmth" factor. This, again, is inferential but observable — more so from direct observation than from a videotape. The mediator should manifest, overtly or covertly, a sense of caring about the child. It is possible to have a mediator who scores high on all other components, but behaves in a rather mechanistic way that communicates indifference or even hostility to the child. On the other hand, it is possible to have a mediator who is very unskilled in many of the components, yet who communicates a strong sense of affection to the child.

Change

Like the component of challenge, the component of change is reserved for application to teachers and assessors because of the time and nature of activity factors. To obtain a high score on this component, it is necessary to articulate the difference between performance prior to and following the interaction, with the implication that the child has profited from the experience. The mediator may need to "reach" for evidence of change, but it is rare that some indication cannot be found.

Reciprocity

Reciprocity is the only component relating to the child's behavior on the MLE Rating Scale. It needs to be scored independently of the mediator's behavior, but any interpretations of mediator behavior should take this component into consideration. Some children, as a result of age and/or temperament factors, make very strong demands on mediators for intentionality and task regulation, for example. It then becomes important to note how a mediator handles this when the demands are made; however, it is also important to note that the demands are being made.

General Comments

One "do" and one "don't" should be added to the comments above. The "do" is to take many notes of the specific behaviors of mediators, especially when the scale is used for diagnostic purposes. The specific way in which a particular mediator expresses each component is as important as the occurrence of the component, and the more idiosyncratic and individual aspects are what provide the basis for discussion and intervention.

The "don't" is to be careful not to be influenced by a positive or negative "halo effect." Each component must be scored independently. A parent who may appear hostile will not necessarily score low on all components; similarly, a parent who appears very verbal and warm will not necessarily have high scores on all the components. If the scale is to be of diagnostic use and a profile generated, each component needs to be considered first separately, and then as part of a configuration.

RESEARCH ON THE MLE ITSELF

Research addressing the MLE *qua* MLE is limited at this time. However, there are two Israeli researchers actively investigating the application of this concept in their studies of parent–child interactions: Pnina S. Klein and David Tzuriel. Klein uses her own scoring of MLE, which is based on a frequency count of each occurrence of five of the components. (Klein has since modified the components included in her scoring, but these are not yet reported in published research; personal communication, 1990.) Tzuriel, whose research in this area is conducted independently of Klein's, uses her method of scoring. One American researcher, Katherine Greenberg, is researching MLE in relation to classroom usage by teachers.

Klein's data are reported in two publications (Klein et al., 1987; Klein, 1988). The 1987 article reports the results of observations of low-SES American mother–child dyads; in this study, mother–child interactions were observed during 10 minutes of free play when the children were 4, 8, 12, 24, 36, and 48 months of age. Her 1988 article reports the results of a study with middle-class Israeli dyads, observed in their homes during feeding, bathing, and free-play episodes when the children were 6, 12, and 24 months of age. The five components of intentionality/reciprocity, transcendence, meaning, competence, and control are included in Klein's definition and scoring of MLE. There are some differences between Klein's and my own definitions of some components, primarily intentionality and meaning.

Interrater reliability is reported for both studies — in fact, for three samples within the two studies. This information is summarized in Table II.1. These data show moderate to high levels of interrater agreement across the three samples, with relative consistency across the samples.

The Klein et al. (1987) study focused on the relationship between MLE and the child's cognitive development, using the Bayley Scales for the younger children and the McCarthy Scales for the older ones. The study also reports frequency of occurrence of the components, as well as stability of the components over the age ranges of the children. The frequency of occurrence of each of the five components showed a significant increase with each increase in age; the components of transcendence, competence, and regulation occurred at very low frequencies across all age ranges for this sample. The components also showed significant stability across all age ranges; the highest levels of stability occurred at ages after 4 months. MLE components did not show a strong relationship with Bayley Scales scores, but were more strongly predictive of later McCarthy Scales scores. MLE at 4 months was not predictive of later performance; most of the MLE components at 24 months were predictive of McCarthy General Cognitive Index

TABLE II.1. Interrater Reliability of Five MLE Components

| Date | *n* (mother–child dyads) | Coefficient ranges | | | | |
		Intentionality/ reciprocity	Transcendence	Meaning	Competence	Control
1987	20 American	>.75	>.75	>.75	>.75	>.75
	40 Israeli	.76–.85	.62–.83	.65–.80	.74–.92	.68–.81
1988	75 Israeli	.72–.91	.59–.84	.63–.87	.71–.92	.55–.87
		($M = .77$)	($M = .80$)	($M = .76$)	($M = .81$)	($M = .74$)

Note. The data are from Klein, Wieder, and Greenspan (1987) and Klein (1988).

(GCI) at 36 months, whereas MLE at 12 months was more strongly predictive of GCI at 48 months. The specific components that were predictive of GCI at later ages were not consistent. Transcendence and control did not become predictive until 24 months; however, this may well relate to the very low frequency of occurrence of these behaviors.

In her 1988 study, Klein found that the frequencies of occurrence for all five MLE components were considerably higher for her middle-class Israeli sample, compared with the previous low-SES sample. There were also higher frequencies during the play as compared with the feeding and bathing situations for this group; the occurrence of mediation during play was particularly high at 24 months. The study also reports substantial intercorrelations among the five components for all age levels and situations. Cross-situational stability was higher at 6 and 12 months, with a reduction at 24 months; feeding and bathing were associated with more consistency. Stability of MLE components across ages was moderately and significantly stable for intentionality/ reciprocity, meaning, and transcendence; competence and control were not consistently stable.

A study by Tzuriel and Eran (1989) included 47 kibbutz children and their mothers, with the ages of the children ranging between 4 years, 7 months and 7 years, 8 months; the dyads were observed for 30 minutes while engaged in free play. This study focused on the relationship between the mothers' MLE and the children's performance on a dynamic and static cognitive measure, as well as the consistency of mothers' MLE between siblings. The dynamic procedure was the Children's Inferential Thinking Modifiability Test (CITM), designed by Tzuriel (see Part I, Chapter 4). The static measure was Raven's Coloured Progressive Matrices, and the MLE scoring was based on Klein's procedure, incorporating the five components indicated above. This study found that the CITM pretest was predicted only by the Raven, whereas the CITM posttest was predicted by the MLE total score and the Raven, and the CITM gain score was predicted only by the MLE total score. The occurrence of transcendence showed a developmental trend (i.e., it was higher for older than for younger siblings). Consistency for siblings was found for the MLE components of competency and regulation (control), and for the MLE total score.

Greenberg (1990) reports preliminary data on her observations of the classroom interactions of teachers from preschool, primary, and secondary levels in Knoxville, Tennessee. These teachers were participating in a study involving a curriculum based on Feuerstein's work, but they were not cognizant of MLE theory at the time of the observations. Scorers were able to maintain interscorer agreement above the 85th percentile. Teachers were scored on evidence of the highest level of occurrence of each component; also, Greenberg's definitions of the components differ somewhat from the present ones, although there is significant overlap, as well as some instances of adoption from the MLE Rating Scale. The percentages of occurrence for each component—abstracted from Greenberg's table reporting the evidence of MLE components in the spontaneous interactions of these teachers with their students, and combining the results across the three levels of schooling—are as follows:

Intent: consistently present, 100%
Responsiveness: consistently present, 100%
Transcendence: domain-specific, high generalization, 47%
Transcendence: general/strategic, reason for use, 4%
Meaning: subjective, more than two occurrences, 52%
Meaning: objective, more than five occurrences, 19%
Competence: task regulation, prompted, 34%
Competence: praise/encouragement, descriptive, 23%
Self-regulation: reason for use, 4%
Goal-directedness: reason for use, 4%; goal and plan, 47%
Reciprocity: all children involved, 90%
Level of thinking elicited (similar to challenge): higher, 69%

Although this list grossly reduces the amount of information offered in the article, and even the full information is preliminary, it can be seen that most of the components (especially those viewed as most specific and central to MLE, and, thereby to metacognitive development) were used at fairly low rates. Such information helps to establish a need for training teachers in how to facilitate cognitive development within the classroom.

RESEARCH ON THE MLE RATING SCALE

My colleagues and I have carried out three studies using the MLE Rating Scale. These studies provide information regarding frequency of occurrence of the components, interrater reliability, internal consistency, cross-situational consistency, and teachability to parents.

One study (Glazier-Robinson, 1986) investigated the relationship between mothers' MLE scores and their children's preschool achievement. This study also provided information regarding interscorer reliability and internal consistency. The subjects were 24 black, low-SES, normally functioning preschool children and their natural mothers. The mothers were asked to play with their children using a standard set of toys, and their 10-minute interactions were videotaped and scored independently by the researchers. Achievement was assessed by Caldwell's Cooperative Preschool Inventory. Interrater reliability is reported for both exact and within-1-point agreement in Table II.2. The table shows moderate to high interrater agreement, ranging from 67% to 100%, with a mean of 82%. Agreement within 1 point was substantial, with a range of 95% to 100% and a mean of 98.5%.

This study found no relationship between MLE and the children's achievement, and a difficult-to-explain negative relationship between MLE and IQ. Among the factors that may have influenced the lack of relationship between IQ and achievement were the narrow range and high level of achievement of this group; their achievement scores were considerably above a level predictable by their IQ scores. In addition, these children were involved in a preschool curriculum that was based on Feuerstein's work, and the mediation they received from this may have interacted with the mediation from their mothers. In a multiple regression, however, the interaction between IQ and MLE accounted for more of the variance of achievement than either variable taken separately. IQ explained 5%, MLE explained 6%, and IQ × MLE explained 13% of the variance.

Table II.3 shows the matrix of intercorrelations among the components of the scale (it should be noted that the version of the scale used in this study was an earlier one). The table shows that each component

TABLE II.2. Exact Reliability (Trials 1 and 2) and Reliability within 1 Point

	Reliability	
Observed behaviors	Exact	± 1 Point
1A. Intentionality	71%	100%
1B. Reciprocity	71%	100%
2. Meaning	96%	100%
3. Transcendence	100%	100%
4A. Competence (task regulation)	71%	95%
4B. Competence (praise and encouragement)	83%	95%
5. Control of behavior	88%	100%
6. Goal-directedness and planning	88%	100%
7. Psychological differentiation	67%	96%
8. MLE (total)	82%	99%

Note. From *The Relationship between Mediated Learning and Academic Achievement* by B. A. Glazier-Robinson, 1986, unpublished master's thesis, Bryn Mawr College. Reprinted by permission of the author.

TABLE II.3. Spearman Correlation Coefficients for Mediated Learning (Whole Group)

Observed behavior	1A	1B	2	3	4A	4B	5	6	7	8
1A. Intentionality	—	.24	.50**	.42*	.53***	.40*	.35	.45*	.80**	.89**
1B. Reciprocity		—	.15	-.04	.31	-.08	.34	.32	.54**	.32
2. Meaning			—	.56**	.38*	.13	-.08	.15	.40*	.54**
3. Transcendence				—	.24	.55**	.06	.11	.42*	.57***
4A. Competence (task regulation)					—	.27	.46*	.50**	.58**	.69***
4B. Competence (praise/encouragement)						—	.18	.29	.57**	.54**
5. Control of behavior							—	.15	.40*	.45*
6. Goal-directedness/planning								—	.58**	.63***
7. Psychological differentiation									—	.84**
8. MLE (total)										—

Note. From *The Relationship between Mediated Learning and Academic Achievement* by B. A. Glazier-Robinson, 1986, unpublished master's thesis, Bryn Mawr College. Reprinted by permission of the author.

$*p < .05.$

$**p < .01.$

contributed significantly to the total score, with the exception of reciprocity. The two components within mediation of competence (task regulation and praise/encouragement) were not significantly related; praise/encouragement showed a relationship with transcendence, whereas task regulation showed relationships with most components. Finally, internal consistency, as determined by Cronbach's alpha, was .83 (Glazier-Robinson, 1986).

Table II.4 provides the data from Glazier-Robinson (1986) showing the mean ratings (range = 0–3) of each of the components for this population. (The components of contingent responsivity and affective involvement were not included at this time.) As in Klein et al.'s (1987) observations of low-SES mothers, the components of transcendence and (in this case, one type of) competence occurred at very low rates. Sharing, which was included in its "shared information" format, was not in evidence.

The second study using the MLE Rating Scale investigated the cross-situational consistency of mothers' MLEs (Lidz, Bond & Dissinger, 1990). This study involved 22 preschool children with their mothers; the families were white and of middle to high SES, with high levels of educational background. Each dyad was videotaped involved in three 10-minute interactions: teaching the child to build a dog with bristle blocks; teaching the child to complete a parquetry picture; and free play with a standard set of toys. The tapes were scored by trained graduate students. Table II.5 provides the mean ratings (range = 0–3) of each of the components for this population.

Table II.5 offers a sample of ratings for a higher-SES population

TABLE II.4. Means and Standard Deviations for Items on the MLE Rating Scale

Item	Mean	SD
1. Intentionality	2.10	0.93
2. Meaning	1.10	1.11
3. Transcendence	0.25	0.53
4. Sharing	—	—
5. Task regulation	2.00	0.91
6. Praise/encouragement	0.75	1.00
7. Control	1.90	0.50
8. Goal-directedness/planning	1.70	0.48
9. Psychological differentiation	1.70	0.93
10. Contingent responsivity	—	—
11. Affective involvement	—	—
12. Reciprocity	2.50	0.66

Note. The data are from Glazier-Robinson (1986).

TABLE II.5. Means, Standard Deviations, and Standard Errors of Measurement for All Items on the MLE Rating Scale

Item[a]	B			P			FP		
	Mean	SE	SD	Mean	SE	SD	Mean	SE	SD
1. Intentionality	2.95	0.04	0.21	2.95	0.04	0.21	2.95	0.04	0.21
2. Meaning	2.59	0.17	0.80	2.54	0.17	0.80	2.82	0.11	0.50
3. Transcendence	1.09	0.25	1.19	0.82	0.20	0.96	1.14	0.20	0.94
4. Sharing	0.86	0.21	0.99	0.50	0.17	0.80	0.73	0.18	0.83
5. Task regulation	2.54	0.11	0.51	2.45	0.17	0.80	2.95	0.04	0.21
6. Praise/ encouragement	1.64	0.16	0.73	1.68	0.21	0.99	1.59	0.18	0.85
7. Control	2.68	0.15	0.72	2.59	0.16	0.73	2.86	0.14	0.64
8. Goal-directedness/ planning	2.59	0.13	0.59	1.86	0.31	1.46	2.00	0.24	1.11
9. Psychological differentiation	2.41	0.16	0.73	2.82	0.11	0.50	2.73	0.12	0.55
10. Contingent responsibility	2.72	0.12	0.55	2.59	0.18	0.85	2.64	0.12	0.58
11. Affective involvement	2.86	0.10	0.47	2.77	0.15	0.68	2.95	0.04	0.21
12. Reciprocity	2.54	0.14	0.67	2.54	0.13	0.60	3.00	0.00	0.00

Note. B, bristle blocks; P, parquetry; FP, free play. From "Consistency of Mother–Child Interaction Using the Mediated Learning Experience (MLE) Scale" by C. S. Lidz, L. Bond, and L. Dissinger, 1990, *Special Services in the Schools, 6,* 145–165. Copyright 1990 by The Haworth Press. Reprinted by permission.

[a]Items are from an earlier version of the MLE Rating Scale and deviate slightly from those in the current, revised version.

than is portrayed in Table II.4. It can be seen that transcendence and praise/encouragement occurred at higher levels for the higher-SES than for the low-SES population, and that sharing, albeit occurring at a very low levels, was in evidence. Many of these subjects scored at the top range in a number of the components. It was rare for these mothers not to obtain the top rating in intentionality, and they showed consistent strength in meaning, task regulation, control, psychological differentiation, contingent responsivity, and affective involvement.

The internal consistency of the scale, as determined by Cronbach's alpha, for this study was .78. Table II.6 shows the correlations of each component with the total score. In this case, all components did not contribute significantly to the total score. The significant contributors included meaning, sharing (shared information), competence (task regulation), competence (praise/encouragement), goal-directedness/ planning, contingent responsivity, and affective involvement. It is

TABLE II.6. Pearson Correlation of Each MLE Item with the Sum of the Other Items

Item[a]	r
1. Intentionality	.16
2. Meaning	.68***
3. Transcendence	.27
4. Sharing	.51*
5. Task regulation	.45*
6. Praise/encouragement	.55**
7. Control	.05
8. Goal-directedness/planning	.57**
9. Psychological differentiation	.41
10. Contingent responsivity	.60**
11. Affective involvement	.64***

Note. Item scores are averaged over the three tasks. From "Consistency of Mother–Child Interaction Using the Mediated Learning Experience (MLE) Scale" by C. S. Lidz, L. Bond, and L. Dissinger, 1990, *Special Services in the Schools, 6,* 145–165. Copyright 1990 by The Haworth Press. Reprinted by permission.

[a]See footnote *a,* Table II.5.

 *$p < .05$.

 **$p < .01$.

 ***$p < .001$.

of interest that the last two components—for this study, new additions—were strong contributors.

Table II.7 shows interrater reliabilities for each component for each of the three situations. The average level of agreement for bristle blocks was .92, for parquetry was .96, and for free play was .89, all highly significant. The table shows moderate to high reliability for most components for most situations. In this case, contingent responsivity, control, and task regulation showed the lowest levels of agreement, varying with the task. Intentionality appears so low because, although the raters agreed in most cases on their highest ratings, they did not disagree in the same direction when they did not assign a 3.

Table II.8 provides the data on intertask consistency. The table shows that the components with the highest consistency were sharing, praise/encouragement, control, contingent responsivity, and affective involvement. Components showing significant agreement across two of the three tasks included meaning and transcendence. The components that showed no consistency included intentionality, task regulation, goal-directedness/planning, and psychological differentiation. The components showing the most consistency have the most to do with interpersonal sensitivity and affect; those also showing some consistency involve induction of abstract thought.

TABLE II.7. Interrater Reliability (Pearson Correlation Coefficients)

Item[a]	B	P	FP	Item average
1. Intentionality	—	—	—	− .09
2. Meaning	.90**	.84**	.90**	.93**
3. Transcendence	.73*	.83**	.85**	.92**
4. Sharing	.74*	.70*	.88**	.85**
5. Task regulation	.66	.81**	.67*	.80**
6. Praise/encouragement	1.00**	.70*	.80**	.95**
7. Control	.38	.77*	—	.48
8. Goal-directedness/planning	.91**	.71*	.10	.76*
9. Psychological differentiation	.81**	—	—	.82**
10. Contingent responsivity	.63	.96**	− .21	.89**
11. Affective involvement	.77*	.75*	1.00**	.90**
12. Reciprocity	.69*	.85**	—	.73*

Note. A dash means that a correlation could not be calculated. B, bristle blocks; P, parquetry; FP, free play. From "Consistency of Mother–Child Interaction Using the Mediated Learning Experience (MLE) Scale" by C. S. Lidz, L. Bond, and L. Dissinger, 1990, *Special Services in the Schools, 6,* 145–165. Copyright 1990 by The Haworth Press. Reprinted by permission.
[a]See footnote *a,* Table II.5.
*$p < .05$.
**$p < .01$.

Finally, in an attempt to take a gross look at the relationship between the MLE of these high-functioning mothers and their high-functioning children, MLE was correlated with the children's scores on the Perceptual–Performance subscale of the McCarthy Scales. These results are shown in Table II.9. With the understanding that virtually all of these children were functioning at a normal or higher level of cognitive development, two components showed a significant relationship with the McCarthy scores: transcendence and reciprocity. Given the limited variance, it is particularly interesting that induction of higher levels of thought showed a relationship with cognitive level. It is also relevant that the receptivity of the child showed a relationship in a negative direction (no child was noncompliant).

In the third study, Glazier-Robinson (1990) addressed the issue of mothers' ability to learn to use MLE with their preschool children. This study included 30 low-SES, mostly black mother–child dyads — 15 in the treatment group (taught MLE) and 15 in the no-treatment group (no exposure to MLE). The mothers in the control group were told that they would be offered the same training following completion of the study (which did occur). These, again, were normally functioning children. The group that was exposed to MLE instruction showed a highly significant increase in their adoption of these components into their play and teaching interactions with their children, at least over the

TABLE II.8. Pearson Correlation between Tasks and the MLE Rating Scale Items

Item[a]	B with P	B with FP	P with FP
1. Intentionality	− .05	− .05	− .05
2. Meaning	.22	.76***	.02
3. Transcendence	.31	.24	.45*
4. Sharing	.63**	.77***	.50*
5. Task regulation	.06	− .20	.41
6. Praise/encouragement	.49*	.59**	.74***
7. Control	.56**	.52**	.48*
8. Goal-directedness/planning	.26	− .07	.00
9. Psychological differentiation	.08	.05	.16
10. Contingent responsivity	.86***	.72***	.55**
11. Affective involvement	.79***	.89***	.90***

Note. B, bristle blocks; P, parquetry; FP, free play. From "Consistency of Mother–Child Interaction Using the Mediated Learning Experience (MLE) Scale" by C. S. Lidz, L. Bond, and L. Dissinger, 1990, *Special Services in the Schools, 6,* 145–165. Copyright 1990 by The Haworth Press. Reprinted by permission.

[a]See footnote *a*, Table II.5.

*$p < .05$.

**$p < .01$.

***$p < .001$.

TABLE II.9. Pearson Correlation of MLE Rating Scale Items with McCarthy Perceptual-Performance Subscale Standard Scores

Item[a]	r
1. Intentionality	− .09
2. Meaning	.13
3. Transcendence	.42*
4. Sharing	.26
5. Task regulation	− .39
6. Praise/encouragement	.23
7. Control	− .29
8. Goal-directedness/planning	.26
9. Psychological differentiation	− .10
10. Contingent responsivity	− .15
11. Affective involvement	.00
12. Reciprocity	− .42*

Note. From "Consistency of Mother–Child Interaction Using the Mediated Learning Experience (MLE) Scale" by C. S. Lidz, L. Bond, and L. Dissinger, 1990, *Special Services in the Schools, 6,* 145–165. Copyright 1990 by The Haworth Press. Reprinted by permission.

[a]See footnote *a*, Table II.5.

*$p < .05$.

short term of this study. This study also showed a positive transfer effect, in that the mothers were taught MLE in relation to a structured teaching situation and spontaneously transferred their use of MLE to a free-play situation. Interrater reliability was quite high, ranging from 83% to 96%.

This concludes the discussion of research on the MLE Rating Scale; the actual scale follows.

MEDIATED LEARNING EXPERIENCE (MLE) RATING SCALE
(for use with parent-child, teacher-child,
examiner-child interactions with preschool children)

Developed by Carol S. Lidz, Psy.D.
Based on the theory and research of Prof. Reuven Feuerstein

Child: _____ Mediator: _____ Task: _____

Rater: _____ Date: _____ Location: _____

1. **INTENTIONALITY:** a conscious attempt by the mediator to influence the behavior of the child. This includes communication to the child of the purpose for the interaction, as well as attempts by the mediator to maintain the child's involvement in the interaction. For children who are already self-regulating and do not require interventions by the mediator to engage them in the activity, rating of intentionality includes the readiness of the mediator to become involved as necessary; therefore, the mediator shows ongoing interest in the activity involvement of the child (in this case, the rating would be a 2, unless a statement of a principle is provided).

   0 = no evidence
   1 = inconsistently present; loses involvement
   2 = consistently in evidence
   3 = in evidence, with statement or encouragement of a principle to induce self-regulation in the child; this principle would apply to the child's ability to maintain attention and inhibit impulsivity

   NOTES:

2. **MEANING:** moving the content from neutral to a position of value and importance; this may be done by affective emphasis or stating that the object or aspect of focus is important and should be noticed (or, vice versa, that it is negative and to be ignored or avoided).

   0 = not in evidence
   1 = calling up labels or concepts already within the child's repertory; saying that it is important and should be noticed (e.g., "Look at this"), but without elaboration
   2 = adding animation or affect to make the activity come alive and provoke interest
   3 = elaboration that expands the information about the activity or object; this elaboration addresses information that is perceptible to the child within the situation

NOTES:

3. **TRANSCENDENCE:** promotion of cognitive bridges between the task or activity and related but not currently present experiences of the child; these may refer to the past or may anticipate the future. These bridges must promote visual images and help to move the child from the perceptual to the conceptual.

> 0 = not in evidence
> 1 = simple, nonelaborated reference to past or future experience
> 2 = elaborated reference
> 3 = elaborated reference includes hypothetical, inferential, or cause-and-effect thinking

NOTES:

4. **SHARING (Joint Regard):** looking and/or commenting on an object of focus initiated by the child. This also includes trying (figuratively or literally) to "see" the activity from the child's point of view—for example, changing posture or making a comment to express empathy and state a feeling or thought that the child might be experiencing. Finally, this also includes statements expressing the "we-ness" of the experience, as in using the term "Let's . . ."; for example: "Wow, that was really hard—we had to work a long time to figure that one out!"

> 0 = not in evidence
> 1 = clear occurrence, but unelaborated reference
> 2 = elaborated reference
> 3 = helping the child express a thought that the child was otherwise unable to elaborate; the expression of the thought should appear to be an accurate reflection of the child's thinking or feeling

NOTES:

5. **SHARING (of Experiences):** communication to the child of an experience or thought the mediator had that the child had not previously shared or experienced with the mediator. Examples: comments including "When I was a little girl . . ." or "This makes me think of . . ."

> 0 = not in evidence
> 1 = clear but nonelaborated reference
> 2 = elaborated reference
> 3 = elaborated reference includes hypothetical, cause-and-effect, or inferential thinking

NOTES:

6. **COMPETENCE** (**Task Regulation**): manipulation of the task to facilitate mastery by the child.

    0 = not in evidence

    1 = simple directions or passive manipulation of the task (e.g., holding it, moving pieces toward the child; building a model without elaborated directions)

    2 = elaborated directions; nonverbal organization into a kind of conceptual grouping

    3 = induction/statement/encouragement of strategic thinking and a planful attitude (e.g., "Where shall we start?" "What should we do first?"), or statement of a principle that the child can use to solve similar problems

NOTES:

7. **COMPETENCE** (**Praise/Encouragement**): verbal or nonverbal communication to the child that he or she did a good job. (Deduct 1 point for negative put-down remarks—i.e., no more than 1 point.)

    0 = not in evidence

    1 = occasional display of nonverbal touch/hug; occasional statement of "Good," "Fine," "Right," etc.

    2 = frequent displays of nonverbal touch/hug; frequent statements of "Good," "Fine," "Right," etc. (frequent = three or more), or encouraging remarks in an attempt to help preserve the child's self-esteem, even if these are not clear praise

    3 = occasional or frequent praise, including information about the child's performance that seems to help the child (e.g., "You really looked at all the choices; that was great!")

NOTES:

8. **COMPETENCE** (**Challenge/Zone of Proximal Development** or ZPD—for application to teachers and examiners; may be omitted for parents for short interactions): maintenance of the activity or task within the child's ZPD (i.e., neither too high nor too low for the child's ability to deal with the task demands); the child should be challenged to reach beyond his or her current level of functioning, but not so overwhelmed as to be discouraged from attempts to engage in the task.

0 = not in evidence; activity is overly frustrating or much too far below the level of challenge

1 = some success in accurate maintenance within ZPD; inconsistently maintained

2 = general success; more in evidence than not

3 = general success, including articulation to the child of the principle that was involved (e.g., "You really had to think and work hard on this, but you were able to do it with only a little help!", or "I want to make this a little hard for you so you have to think, but I'll give you some help so you will know what to do," or "This is too hard to do it by yourself—can I teach it to you?")

NOTES:

9. **PSYCHOLOGICAL DIFFERENTIATION:** maintenance of the idea that the role of the mediator is to facilitate the learning of the child, not to have a learning experience for himself or herself (at this time). Thus, there should be no indications of competitiveness with the child or of rejecting of the child's efforts to engage in the task. The focus of the mediator is on provision of a good learning experience rather than on creation of a good product; if something has to be sacrificed, it is the end product, not the child's experience. (Deduct 1 point if the mediator rejects the child's efforts to become involved.)

0 = not in evidence; mediator poorly differentiated

1 = activity is mostly mediator's, only occasionally the child's

2 = activity is mostly child's, with only occasional lapses by the mediator

3 = activity is clearly and consistently child's, with mediator maintaining an objective, facilitating role

NOTES:

10. **CONTINGENT RESPONSIVITY:** ability to read the child's cues and signals related to learning, affective, and motivational needs, and then to respond in a timely and appropriate way.

0 = not in evidence

1 = infrequent, inconsistent (ill timed or not appropriate)

2 = present, but occasionally missing the mark either in timing or in appropriateness

3 = consistently well timed and appropriate to child's cues and signals

NOTES:

11. **AFFECTIVE INVOLVEMENT:** communication of a sense of caring about and enjoyment of the child; this may be overt or more quietly covert, but it should be clear that there is a feeling of joy in the child's presence, with signs of emotional attachment. This should appear more strongly in a parent than in a teacher or examiner, but should be in evidence in any of the mediators.

    0 = not in evidence; indifferent; may be negative
    1 = minimal evidence; neutral, but not negative or indifferent
    2 = clear evidence; may have lapses
    3 = clear and consistent enjoyment

NOTES:

12. **CHANGE** (for application to teachers and examiners): communication to the child that he or she has profited in a positive direction from the experience — that he or she has improved and changed in some way, compared to the starting point. This includes providing the child with actual pre–post product comparisons, as well as pre–post behavioral descriptions.

    0 = not in evidence
    1 = weak evidence
    2 = strong, but unelaborated evidence
    3 = strong indications, including elaborated feedback regarding what the child did and what the changes were; these might also include elicitations from the child regarding what he or she notices has changed

NOTES:

SCORE SEPARATELY AND DO NOT INCLUDE IN MLE TOTAL, BUT INCLUDE FOR ALL SITUATIONS:

RECIPROCITY OF CHILD: the level of receptivity of the child to the mediational intentions of the adult. How open is the child to input from the mediator? How able or willing to "receive" or cooperate?

    0 = highly resistant; mediation cannot effectively proceed
    1 = minimally receptive; frequent resistance
    2 = moderately receptive; occasional lapses
    3 = consistently receptive and cooperative

NOTES:

PROFILE OF MEDIATOR FUNCTIONING ON THE MEDIATED LEARNING EXPERIENCE RATING SCALE

	3	2	1	0
1. Intentionality				
2. Meaning				
3. Transcendence				
4. Sharing (joint regard)				
5. Sharing (of experiences)				
6. Task regulation				
7. Praise/encouragement				
8. Challenge				
9. Psychological differentiation				
10. Contingent responsivity				
11. Affective involvement				
12. Change				

Child's Responsivity:

Summary:

APPENDIX II.A. Sample Home Activities

ACTIVITY 1

COGNITIVE FUNCTION: Planning
"When we have a lot to do, it helps to make a plan."
1. Determining what is needed to do the task
2. Determining what the best order is, and if the order matters
3. Deciding on special strategies
4. Evaluating the effectiveness of the plan

ACTIVITY: Making a salad
Type of salad:

MATERIALS NEEDED:
Ingredients:
Utensils:

PROCEDURE:
Getting started (Intentionality)
1. Decide what you need to make the salad. You might say to your child something like this: "Let's make a _____ salad to eat. I can use your help. Can you help me figure out what we need?"
2. Think about the best order for the steps needed to make your salad, and reasons for this order. Talk with your child about this. You might say, "Now we have all the things we need. What do we need to do first? Why is that a good idea? What would happen if we did something else first? Does it matter?"

    Things to think about: When does order make a difference?
        a. Does it make sense to wash, peel, and then cut the vegetables?
        b. Does it matter which ingredient goes in first?
        c. What is the best organization for the task? How can you divide up the work?

Making it interesting (Meaning)
1. Talk about what you are doing with interest and emotion. Consider the ingredients in terms of their color, shape, texture, taste, and so on. You might ask your child questions such as these: "What color is the _____? What shape is it? How does it feel?"
2. Expand the possibilities of what can be done. For example, you might say something like this: "This time we cut the carrots into circle shapes. Maybe next time we can cut them a different way."

3. Give explanations for why things are done in a particular way. For example, you might say, "The knife is sharp and could cut you, so we need to be very careful and hold it this way."

Bridging to past and future thinking (Transcendence)
1. Discuss with your child how planning helped with this activity. You might ask questions such as these: "Did it help to do things in order? Can you think of anything else you might need to plan? What about getting dressed in the morning? What plan can we make for that?"
2. Talk about how the food in the salad helps us to grow to be healthy. For example, you might tell your child, "Carrots help us to see better."

Applying what we learn to other things (Generalization)
1. Later, perhaps at dinner, have your child recall what you did together, what you noticed and learned about the activity, and how it helped to make a plan. Help your child to remember the order followed for the salad.
2. Encourage your child to tell someone else about making the salad.
3. Plan another cooking time together. What else can you make?

ACTIVITY 2

COGNITIVE FUNCTION: Comparing
1. Noticing how things are the same and different
2. Learning to follow a model
3. Learning what to notice when looking at a model

ACTIVITY: Matching pictures from a magazine

MATERIALS NEEDED:
1. Comfortable place to sit
2. Magazine with many colorful pictures
   Name of magazine:
   Pictures chosen for matching:

PROCEDURE:
Getting started (Intentionality)
1. Plan a time when you will have 15 to 20 minutes alone with your child. You might say, "Let's look at this magazine together. I think you will like this one; it has many pretty pictures to look at. Where can we sit together?" Encourage your child to sit on your lap, if your child will accept that, or to lean against you with your arm around him or her.

2. As you look through the magazine, find a picture that might be of interest to your child, or let your child find one that is of interest. Name the picture and describe some of its features; make sure you sound interested. Then say, "Let's find another one like this. What shall we look for?" When another one within the same category is located, say, "Yes, these are both _____ . How is this one like the first one? How are they different?" You may need to guide your child with some ideas. For example: "Do you see something that looks the same? Is there something about the color that might be the same? Is there something about the shape?"

3. Find other items in the magazine for which you can find similar matches. Compare these and discuss how they are the same and different. You can try naming a feature of the model picture (e.g., "This one has dots; does the other one have dots? No? Then they are different because one has dots and the other has stripes"), and then ask your child to check the second picture to see whether it has the same thing.

Making it interesting (Meaning)

1. Talk about what you are doing with interest. Try to discover what your child finds interesting about the picture. Say things like "That's funny! That's neat! That's strange! I like that!"

2. Show some excitement when you speak.

3. Elaborate on the picture you select; tell your child at least one thing about it — something like this: "These shoes don't look comfortable. They look like they would hurt. The toes are so pointy."

4. Try to make your discussion and time together game-like. Think of a fun way to say things, such as "Simon Says. . . ."

Bridging to past and future (Transcendence)

1. Ask your child to think of something you have in your home that is like the item in the picture. Talk about how that item is similar to or different from the item in the picture.

2. Ask your child this: "If you could have an item something like the one in the picture, what would it be like? What would you do with it?"

Applying what we learn (Generalization)

1. Later in the day, have your child recall what you looked at in the magazine.

2. Encourage your child to tell someone else about the things you saw and discussed.

3. Talk about other items you have in the house (e.g., fruit, vegetables, furniture, clothing, toys, etc.). Ask your child to describe one of these. Then ask your child to think of another item something like that, and discuss how they are the same or different.

4. When you go to the supermarket and have to buy more than one item of a certain type, pick one out and have your child find another one. Talk about how they are the same or different: "Oh, that's even bigger!" "Look, this one is very bumpy."

5. Draw an outline of a picture of something from the magazine. Ask your child to color in the outline to look as much like the picture as possible. (Be sure to make it simple enough so it can be done.)

6. Plan another activity where you and your child can compare.

III

MANUAL FOR THE PRESCHOOL LEARNING ASSESSMENT DEVICE AND FOR A CURRICULUM-BASED ADAPTATION

INTRODUCTION

This manual describes both a "generic" dynamic assessment approach developed for use with young children that draws most consistently from Feuerstein's model, and a curriculum-based adaptation of this approach. These procedures attempt a downward, but not a literal, extension of Feuerstein's model for use with preschool children from the ages of 3 through 5 years, although the curriculum-based procedure may well be usable with children throughout their school-age years.

Any assessment procedure must include at least three elements, and this applies to dynamic assessment as well. These elements include a way to describe the learner (i.e., what is to be noted, observed, recorded, and addressed regarding the learner's behavior?), a way to describe the assessor (what is the assessor to do during the course of the assessment?), and a way to describe the task (to what types of tasks do these results generalize?). Both the "generic" Preschool Learning Assessment Device (PLAD) and the curriculum-based adaptation are based on a model that addresses these issues as follows. The learner is described in terms of a theory of cognitive functioning related to the Luria-based "planning–arousal–simultaneous–successive" (PASS) model elaborated by Naglieri and Das (1988), which is discussed below. This theory is then extended into a listing and operationalization of cognitive processes that serve as the specific targets of intervention, as well as a means for describing the child as learner. The assessor's behavior is described in terms of my adaptation of Feuerstein's concept of the Mediated Learning Experience (MLE), followed by an elaborated listing of an array of educational interventions that sample the "best practices" education literature available to date. The concept of MLE provides a global description of interactional processes that should be occurring during the course of the assessment, whereas the list of specific interventions constitutes the elaboration of the more general concepts of such items as "meaning," "transcendence," and "task regulation." The guidelines for the provision of MLE are operationalized by the MLE Rating Scale, described in Part II of this text. Finally, the tasks and task components are described both in terms of content and in terms of cognitive demands, so that it is possible to determine expectations for generalization of assessment results. These are describable in terms of a modification of Feuerstein's cognitive map.

This manual also provides information regarding how to record, interpret, and report the results obtained with both the PLAD and the curriculum-based adaptation, as well as the research results available to date. The research on dynamic assessment in general and on this model in particular is very limited, and no claim is made that there is sufficient data to support either the validity or reliability of the model. The procedures are presented here in experimental form, with the intent to encourage further research and investigation.

Users who are new to dynamic assessment procedures may at first perceive more similarity between these and psychometric measures than is really the case. This approach to dynamic assessment is extremely challenging for assessors, since there is considerable demand for "on-the-spot" analysis of the learner, and quick decisions are necessary to determine appropriate interventions. While all these processes are going on, the assessor must also record events and keep in mind the need to carry out the basic tenets of an MLE. Needless to say, this cannot be easily gleaned from simply reading a manual. Supervised practice is essential to adequate mastery. This is a clinical procedure that involves some clinical inference; such clinical skill is viewed as a positive value of this approach, rather than a source of embarrassment. The fact that the procedure is clinical and inferential does not take away from the need to demonstrate reliability of conclusions derived from its implementation, but there will never be a way to conduct an item analysis or even to determine intratest consistency, since not every assessor will be behaving in exactly the same way at the same time. The results of this assessment should, however, show validity in terms of recommendations for instruction that result in successful learning, if the recommendations from the assessment are implemented.

It should be glaringly clear that test–retest stability is incompatible with the concept of dynamic assessment, and in fact would indicate procedural invalidity. If the procedure does not produce change, then either the interventions selected were not appropriate, or insufficient time was available to induce the desired effects. The weight is on the assessor to find a way to reach the child, rather than on the child to demonstrate competency to the assessor. It should not be possible to conclude that a child is untestable or unteachable — only that it has not yet been possible to find the means to help the child profit from experience. There is no presumption here that all children are capable of normal levels of functioning; it is only presumed that all children are capable of some degree of change. The extent of this change can only be estimated by a child's actual response to attempts to induce change, and one value underlying this approach to assessment is that there is no *a priori* assumption about the capacities of children — certainly none dictated exclusively by IQ.

Some of the outcomes of this approach to dynamic assessment have already been mentioned, but they can be summarized briefly here. Dynamic assessment should inform us of the following:

1. The child's degree of responsivity to intervention (i.e., the types of interventions provided during the course of the assessment).

2. The intensity of intervention required to produce these changes.

3. A descriptive profiling of the child's cognitive strengths and weaknesses, in terms of the types of tasks and interventions provided.

4. Hypotheses regarding the types of interventions that promote or obstruct success.

Previous attempts to design dynamic assessments have been more successful in their attempts to describe the learner and to demonstrate responsiveness of the learner to intervention than in deriving linkages to classroom intervention procedures. This model of dynamic assessment, particularly in its curriculum-based adaptation, is an attempt to link psychoeducational assessment with the instructional setting. Such a linkage has never been successfully accomplished by psychometric batteries. Although curriculum-based approaches have proved promising, even these procedures lack information about the child as learner. There is no intent here to dismiss either psychometric or curriculum-based approaches as useless or lacking in meaning. Rather, as assessors, we need to be aware of the types of information any of our procedures provides, and to acknowledge that procedures designed for one purpose cannot necessarily be successfully employed for another for which they were never intended.

This model of dynamic assessment is designed as an addition to the assessment repertory. Information is provided that responds to questions that other procedures are not designed to address. If we wish to determine how far the child's knowledge base deviates from the norm, we will continue to administer a psychometric measure. If we wish to determine the content of the child's knowledge base within a specific domain, we will administer a curriculum-based or criterion-referenced test. If we wish to derive hypotheses about how the child learns, how responsive the child is to attempts to intervene, and what seems to be interfering with the child's ability to profit from existing attempts at instruction, we will use dynamic assessment. Dynamic assessors first need to be astute clinicians; dynamic assessment procedures are perhaps the least assessor-proof of all available approaches. We need to learn more about how to select and develop good assessors, just as we need to learn more about how to develop good parents and teachers. The fact that this is necessary should not induce us to dismiss the procedure, but should stimulate our efforts to improve training.

Although this model represents yet another instance of focusing on the child, the model presents no contradiction to the need to proceed with any assessment in terms of an ecologically valid perspective. In fact, the elaboration of MLE provides a means of looking at significant aspects of the child's ecology — namely, assessors, teachers, and parents. The model also forces assessors to consider in great detail the elements of the task as a primary variable. Again, this model represents another piece of the assessment picture, not its entirety. The procedures do not replace the need to include other measures such as interviews and observations that address other components of the child's ecology. With all this in mind, welcome to the world of dynamic assessment!

THEORETICAL BASIS

Assessment procedures may be either empirically derived or theoretically based. Those that are empirically derived are typically concerned with discrimination among groups; that is, the procedures are based on the fact that they discriminate between, for example, good and poor learners. Not only is there an increased attempt to base assessment procedures on theory, but in the case of dynamic assessment this is especially necessary, since the approach is not intended for use as a psychometrically discriminating instrument. Theoretical bases for assessments allow both forward and backward reasoning regarding the meaning and interpretation of results. In the case of dynamic assessment, it is desirable to be able to conclude that the results reveal important information about the learning process, and it is equally desirable to derive the details of the procedure from a conceptualization of the learning process. The components of the assessment should reflect aspects of cognition that are speculated (or, preferably, demonstrated) to relate to the teaching–learning process, and that allow the linkage between the assessment results and the child's functioning as a learner in the classroom.

The theory base for this dynamic assessment approach and for the MLE Rating Scale (see Part II) derives primarily from Luria (1966,

1973), as elaborated by Naglieri and Das (1988), Vygotsky (1978, 1988), and Feuerstein (1979, 1980). The need is to derive a basis for determination of the cognitive processes relevant to the educational enterprise that can be used to describe both the learner and the assessor. Critics of so-called "process" approaches to assessment and intervention seem to imply that it is sufficient simply to identify the content of what needs to be learned, and to expose the child to this content. Such a simplistic approach ignores the children who fail to profit from instruction. We must be able to identify what is making a specific learning episode difficult for the child, and to derive approaches to facilitate the child's competence. If the solution is merely to simplify the task or to provide more practice, then a dynamic assessment is unlikely to be necessary. A dynamic assessment is relevant for children who do not respond to the "usual" teaching practices; in these cases, it is necessary to obtain a more in-depth understanding of what seems to be going wrong. At times, the answer may require finding the optimal manipulation of the task variables; at other times, the answer may relate to the way a child processes or fails to employ strategies in relation to the task. In order to discover the variables that result in development of competence for the child, it is necessary to have an idea of what to look for in the child's functioning in relation to task demands, and it is here that our theories can provide guidance.

The theoretical basis, as elaborated here, is intended to provide a foundation for meaningful conceptualization of the dynamic assessment procedure, and is not intended to represent a sophisticated interpretation of human neuropsychological functioning. Concepts developed to describe and explain neuropsychological functions have been abstracted, reduced, and interpreted in terms of their relationships to the educational interaction and their implications for the teaching (as mediation)–learning process. Thus, the theories are used to the extent that they promote understanding of the educational endeavor, rather than understanding of the neurological foundations for learning.

Luria's theories explicating the neuropsychological foundations of thinking provide the foundations for understanding thinking as a dynamic, active, and integrated process. Vygotsky's conceptualization of the mediating role of the socializing agents portrays this important source of environmental stimuli as similarly dynamic and active. Thus, the relevance of the term "dynamic" for the assessment approach described here becomes obvious. The question of what is "dynamic" about dynamic assessment is answerable in terms of the processes addressed and the interventions with which these processes are mediated. These concepts contrast with formulations of teaching, learning, and thinking processes as static or passive.

It is important to be reminded that not every situational interaction of the learner involves thinking. The nature of the dynamic assessment situation is to set up the conditions for thinking to occur, to assess the degree to which thinking is in evidence, and to induce the occurrence of thinking in relation to the tasks presented. What Luria, Vygotsky, Feuerstein, and others are discussing are the characteristics of thinking and the extent to which these characteristics can be assessed and promoted in the learner.

An additional advantage to basing this procedure on the theories of Luria and on the Naglieri and Das (1988) PASS model is the potential for closer linkage between a psychometric and a dynamic approach, so that one can flow more naturally from the other during the course of the assessment. It is likely that the question of determining the current levels of functioning of the child in relation to peers will remain a viable assessment issue. The PASS model is an attempt to improve upon our current approaches to psychometric determination of cognitive status. It would appear useful, then, to be able to move from the normative estimation of where the child is currently functioning in relation to his peer group to an estimation of how fixed the child is in that normative relationship, as well as to link this normative information with intervention hypotheses for the child who is dysfunctional. Having both the psychometric and dynamic assessment approaches derived from the same theoretical base makes a good deal of sense in promoting such consistency, given that the theoretical base is demonstrated to be a valid representation of the processes it purports to describe and explain.

Why Process?

Given the frustrating history of the search for the "real" processes that matter in education, it is relevant to ask a question at this point: "Why are we focusing on process (yet again) in relation to classroom learning, especially in view of the growing popularity of such approaches as curriculum-based assessment?" The response is deceptively simple. If we ask questions such as "How do children learn?" "Why do children fail to learn?" and "How can children best be taught?", the answers necessarily involve process. The response to why a referred child is not learning to decode reading cannot be that the child is not able to decode reading, or that the child is currently reading at a preprimer level.

The need to consider process is well illustrated by the relatively recent research involving the study of intelligence in infancy. It is a well-known finding that the results of infant assessments are poor predictors of later cognitive development for all but those who clearly function at a deficient level. Much stronger predictions of later development have emerged from studies involving attention, habituation, and parenting interactions (i.e., processes). Also, researchers such as Naglieri, Das, and Jarman (1990) are increasingly criticizing traditional psychometric measures of cognitive functioning for failing to tap processes relevant to learning and processes that show promise of discriminating between groups of learners. These authors provide evidence that Luria-based processes show meaningful differences between groups with various disadvantages or deficiencies (e.g., reading disability, attention deficits, delinquency) and normals. Furthermore, dynamic assessment and its related interventions set the goal of developing learners who are active and self-regulating (i.e., able to direct and monitor their own learning). This again necessitates consideration of process.

In my view, assessment developers, perhaps out of justified frustration with the history of the poor match between assessment and instruction, have become overfond of content in a time of continuing content/information explosion. Such focus on content lacks implications both for teaching and for diagnosing learner response. Knowing only what the learner does or does not know, or at what level she knows, may accurately locate the next instructional step; however, it offers nothing to inform the accomplishment of the instructional objective — that is, unless we posit a strictly associationistic model, which then suggests that practice and drill are the preferred teaching modalities for all instances. Although the importance of content and the need to develop a solid knowledge base (even, in some circumstances, to the point of automaticity) cannot be denied, dynamic assessment is based on a further concern with development of the ability to self-regulate and to self-determine what needs to be done and how in any specific learning situation. An associationistic point of view generates dependence on the stimulus supplier, and is antithetical to self-regulation and active learning. A more cognitive/process-oriented viewpoint moves the learner into shared responsibility for stimulation and may even be viewed as more relevant to democratic values than is the more autocratic, associationistic, behavioristic model. Thus, the processes that become most relevant for a "dynamic" learner are those most often associated with metacognition (e.g., determination and application of relevant strategies, self-evaluation, self-monitoring), as well as those that reflect psychological manifestations of our most basic yet malleable neurological functions (e.g., attention, memory, strategic thinking). It is difficult for anyone to deny that processes such as attention and memory are important for learning. However, these are rarely the primary foci of assessment, and despite the increasing research evidence to support the relevance of metacognitive processes to learning, there is even less attention to these processes in our traditional assessment approaches. These constitute the primary foci of dynamic assessment.

Which Processes?

Determination of the specific processes to be assessed provides an operationalization of the "learner" in the triad of the learner, the assessor, and the task, which comprise the basic components of any assessment system. The issue here is this: What is it we wish to notice and to record about the learner? It is then assumed that these form the basis for what is to be "modified" — what is to be profiled in terms of strengths and weaknesses, and what is to be addressed by specific intervention strategies. These processes also provide a basis for one aspect of the task analysis, as each task is viewed in terms of its process demands. Thus, there is an exact match between the demands of the task and the functioning of the learner, since both are described in exactly the same manner.

The Basic Model

The primary model for derivation of processes in this approach to dynamic assessment is the "planning–arousal–simultaneous–successive" (PASS), Luria-based model described by Naglieri, Das, and colleagues (Naglieri & Das, 1988; Naglieri, 1989; Naglieri et al., 1990). These authors describe a nonlinear, dynamically interactive input–elaboration–output model of mental activity derived from Luria's neurologically based observations and research, as well as from the results of their own numerous investigations. The model includes three major functional units that are involved in mental activity. These are "arousal/attention," which involves maintenance of an optimal state of arousal and facilitation of voluntary attention mechanisms (discussed in terms of selective, sustained, and divided attention); "coding," which is made up of simultaneous ("each element of the stimuli is interrelated to every other element") and successive ("integration of stimuli into a specific sequential series, where each element is related only to the next") integrative processes, with each of these processes applicable to perceptual and memory (storage and retrieval) functions; and, finally, "planning" ("acts to organize the individual's conscious activity once information has been received, coded, and stored so that the individual can form plans of action, inspect the performance and regulate behavior so that it conforms to these plans"). (All quotations are from Naglieri & Das, 1988, pp. 37–38.) The planning function involves formulation of an action plan, carrying out of the plan (requiring self-regulation), and evaluation of the effectiveness of the plan (with consequent adjustment). Any specific task or activity has content that is perceived, analyzed, coded, and stored, and this content is referred to as the "knowledge base." Finally, there is an "output" aspect of mental processing, which is not elaborated upon here.

Each of the processes has distinct neurological correlates, although all act together to define mental processing. The arousal function is in evidence throughout the mental activity and should be in evidence in relation to any type of activity. Tasks differ primarily in their coding demands (whether simultaneous or successive). Regardless of the type of coding required, the processes of perception/acquisition and storage/retrieval apply. The planning function may influence any of the coding functions and may relate to the success with which these are carried out — for example, reflecting the learner's ability to evaluate the types of strategies required for the type of task, to apply these to the task, and to evaluate their effectiveness. Naglieri (1989) and Naglieri and Das (1988) offer evidence to support the existence of these processes and have developed a series of tasks for their psychometric assessment procedure, en route to their attempt to devise an alternative approach to assessment of intelligence.

The major units of this model form the basis of the recording format to be employed during the course of the dynamic assessment procedure, whether this is applied to preschool or to older (school-age) children. This format appears in Appendix III.A. In this format, the task demands first need to be analyzed, and this is done in terms of an adaptation of Feuerstein's (1979, 1980) cognitive map, which appears in Appendix III.B. As the assessor works with the learner, observations are recorded to indicate the extent to which the necessary processes and knowledge base are present in the learner, and the degree to which these are responsive to the interventions offered. More detailed operational definitions of processes, and examples of types of interventions, are offered below.

THE BASIC MODEL ELABORATED: TARGETS OF ASSESSMENT

In this section, each process to be addressed in the assessment is defined, the mediational interventions to be utilized during the course of the assessment are discussed, and additional interventions applicable to the classroom situation are offered. These processes and interventions apply to any type of dynamic assessment that incorporates the model offered here (i.e., these are not specific to the PLAD or its curriculum-based adaptation).

The theory and components of the MLE to be offered during the assessment by the assessor have been elaborated in greater detail in Part II, which describes the MLE Rating Scale. The nature of the intervention stage of the test–intervene–retest assessment model is to provide an optimal MLE. Some of the MLE components are individualized in terms of their relationship to specific processes; however, many are general, applicable to all processes, and not so readily customized. I have adopted most of the components described by Feuerstein (1979, 1980), but have made some additions in response to literature reviews of the relationship between parent–child interactions and cognitive development. The specific definitions reflect my interpretations and adaptations of Feuerstein's original components.

The general MLE components include mediation of the following: intentionality; two aspects of sharing (shared focus and sharing of experience); two aspects of competence (praise/encouragement, and challenge in terms of maintenance within the child's zone of proximal development [ZPD]); psychological differentiation; contingent responsivity; affective involvement; and change. All of these are offered in terms of responsivity to the child's level of reciprocity, in addition to functioning to optimize the child's reciprocity. "Reciprocity" is defined as the extent to which the child is willing to cooperate with the interaction, and the extent to which the child is able to "receive" (process) the mediation from the assessor. The MLE components that are customized include mediation of meaning, transcendence, and a third aspect of competence (task regulation).

Feuerstein's components of control/regulation and of goal seeking, setting, and planning are not included here as separate MLE components, because of the reworking of the theory in terms of Luria's conceptualization, which places attention (control/regulation) and planning in the category of processes characteristic of the learner. Thus, these components become targets within the child addressed by the mediation. The ultimate criterion for optimal mediation of any component is the extent to which it promotes self-regulated, active learning in the child; therefore, any attempt at mediation that offers or reinforces a principle that the child can internalize and apply to a broader range of situations than the immediate task or portion of the task is rated more highly than is a specific directive. Also, all mediation is evaluated in terms of the extent to which it induces development and utilization of metacognitive processes characteristic of the planning functions; it is assumed that such utilization facilitates self-regulation and impulse control in the learner. Therefore, the goal-directedness/ planning and control/self-regulation aspects of the components have been incorporated as elements of all components to define their optimal occurrence. These changes are rationalized in terms of their contribution toward increasing the discreteness of the categories, and thus facilitating their clarity for scoring and training purposes.

Mediation is conceptualized here as what the assessor does. Processes such as attention and memory are functions targeted for modification within the learner. The ongoing and ultimate objective of mediation is to induce the application of metacognitive strategies in relation to the process of focus, thereby enhancing the learner's ability to self-regulate and become an active participant in the learning process. Thus, mediation of task regulation, for example, when applied either to attention or to coding processes, will aim to induce self-regulation via induction of planning processes. In this way the model becomes less linear and more interactive and dynamic, as intended by Luria's representation of mental activity.

General Components of MLE (Assessor Behaviors)

The general components of MLE are reviewed here; the reader is referred to the MLE Rating Scale manual in Part II for further details and elaborations.

1. *Intentionality.* Demonstrations of intent by the mediator represent a conscious attempt to influence the behavior of the child. That is, the idea is communicated to the child that the assessor is here for a specific purpose. It is anticipated that few assessors or teachers will have difficulty with this component, although some parents do. Manifestations of intent include informing the child of the purpose for the interaction, as in this example: "We are here to work together to find the best ways to teach you in school. I noticed that in the work we have done so far, you had some difficulty with [specify processes to be addressed]. These sometimes make learning in school hard for you. Today we are going to try to figure out how to help you be a good learner." Thus, statements of the goal and purpose of the interaction are included in intentionality. Intent is then continued by remaining in the role of an active intervener who maintains engagement in the process of conscious influence throughout the interaction. Intentionality is also involved when the mediator works to maintain or regain the child's involvement with the task. At its highest, "planning" level, intentionality elicits or offers strategies for self-control or self-regulation, including offering a principle that the child can potentially

internalize for self-regulation. For example: "Can you get yourself ready to pay attention? Good! You are sitting up straight and looking right at me," or, "I notice that you really need to stand up every once in a while to help you pay attention better; would you like to try that?"

2. *Sharing (shared focus).* Sharing in terms of shared focus or joint regard occurs when the mediator looks and comments on an initiation of the child, when the mediator tries (figuratively or literally) to "see" the task from the child's point of view, and when the mediator expresses the "we-ness" of the learning interaction. This includes comments such as "Let's figure out how we can do this," or empathic statements that attempt to reflect and express the child's reactions, such as "Wow, that was a hard one, wasn't it?" Other illustrations of sharing include physical positioning by the mediator in a literal attempt to "see" the task from the child's point of view. Shared focus at its highest or planning level involves an attempt by the mediator to infer and elaborate some thoughts or feelings that the child may be having in relation to the task. For example, the mediator might say, "I was wondering if you were afraid to try that because it looked so hard."

3. *Sharing (sharing experiences).* Sharing of experience occurs when the mediator communicates to the child an experience related to the task or situation that the mediator had that the child has not shared with the mediator. This has the potential effect of broadening the child's repertory of information, of allowing the mediator to join and relate to the child's experience, and of promoting the child's internalization of learning by means of identification with the mediator. Sharing may have the secondary effects of enhancement of meaning and of promoting transcendence, but the primary element is the "joining" effect between mediator and child. Sharing of experience at its highest, or planning, level offers some abstract concept involving cause-and-effect or hypothetical thinking relating to the mediator's experiences. For example: "You know, when I saw these blocks it made me remember trying to build things with my brother and how I had to try to think of something he would like to build."

4. *Competence (praise/encouragement).* Mediation of competence by means of providing praise and encouragement includes verbal and/or nonverbal indications to the child that he did a good job and, by inference, is a competent learner. In its most optimal form, statements of praise include feedback to the child about what she did that was so effective or good. For example, while statements of "Good!" or "Great!" are positive instances and promote good feelings, a statement such as "See, you kept trying even though it was hard. Now look at what a good job you did!" is rated more highly because it provides a self-regulating

principle that the child can potentially internalize and apply to other situations (viz., "Persistence may promote success").

5. *Competence (challenge by maintenance within the child's ZPD).* This aspect of mediation of competence (there are a total of three such aspects) involves regulation of the difficulty level of the task presentation, so that on the one hand the child is challenged and encouraged to reach beyond his current level of functioning, while on the other hand the child is not overwhelmed and unduly frustrated. This component relates to mediation of competence via task regulation and to the separate component of contingent responsivity, but represents the ability of the mediator to provide flexible management of the task presentation so that it remains an optimal match for the child. How the mediator does this is a matter of task regulation, and the degree to which it is responsive in timing is a matter of contingent responsivity; the fact that it remains a good match and the outcome is within the child's ZPD is the critical aspect of this component. Thus, it is possible for the mediator to be providing many types of task regulation, even with general self-regulation-promoting principles; however, the mediator may still not be optimizing the match so that the child can attain mastery and achieve competence. Regulation of competence via mediation of challenge occurs at the highest, or planning, level when the mediator explicitly articulates what she is trying to accomplish — that is, to regulate the task for the child so that the child is challenged and not frustrated. For example: "I'm trying to figure out how to make this interesting for you, but not so hard that you don't like it."

6. *Psychological differentiation.* As is true of the component of intentionality, psychological differentiation is a component with which few assessors or teachers experience difficulty, whereas many parents do not do well with this. This component involves maintenance of the idea that the role of the mediator is to facilitate the learning of the child, not to have a learning experience for himself. Thus, there should be no indications of competing with the child, rejecting the child's efforts to engage in the task, setting up parallel tasks, or taking the task away from the child (all of which have been observed in some parental interactions). The mediator demonstrates concern with the process of learning and the fact that the child needs to profit from the experience, rather than with the appearance of the final product.

7. *Change.* The component of mediation of change is one that is frequently missing from teaching interactions. This involves the communication to the child that she has indeed profited from the experience, that she has shown herself to be a learner, and that her final product and behaviors are in some meaningful way different from her

starting products and behaviors. This includes providing the child with pre–post comparisons of what she produced before and after the intervention. Even in the event of minimal (or barely perceptable) change, it is usually possible to find some evidence of modifiability; this is overtly communicated to the child, with the implied message that "Yes, you are a learner; you are modifiable." Mediation of change at the highest, or planning, level involves explicit articulation of not only the fact of change, but inclusion of details regarding the way(s) in which the learner has proved to be modifiable.

8. *Contingent responsivity.* A mediator who is contingently responsive is able to read the child's cues and signals related to learning, affective, and motivational needs and to respond in a timely and appropriate way. This occurs at the highest, or planning, level when there is optimal timing and optimally appropriate response, so that the child experiences predictable, positive, and accurate reactions to his actions and is able to derive feelings of being able to produce a response that can be cognitively anticipated.

9. *Affective involvement.* Although the affective involvement of a school-based assessor is expected to differ from the affective involvement of a parent as mediator, it is nevertheless proposed that a mediator who communicates a sense of caring about and enjoyment of the child will promote greater success in learning than one who is affectless, and certainly more than one who is negativistic or punitive. This is more of a general contextual variable and cannot be elaborated in terms of planning or metacognitive implications.

These, then, are the components of MLE that apply across all processes and tasks. It is proposed that when an optimal MLE is taking place, all of these will be in evidence somewhere during the course of an extended interaction, and that the presence of these components (including those that will be delineated with greater individualization as related to specific processes) will facilitate the child's cognitive development and ability to profit from instruction.

Mediation is interpreted in this model as behaviors engaged in by the teaching or parenting adult that have the potential to influence the child's cognitive processes. Good mediation should promote good learning. Conversely, when deficiencies of learning are observed, it should be possible to evaluate not only the presence or absence of processing components in the learner, but the presence or absence of mediational components in the teaching adult. In this case, learning ability is not conceptualized as restricted to IQ, but is defined in terms of responsiveness to instruction/intervention and in terms of conceptual adaptability to challenge and novelty, combined with level-of-performance indicators such as IQ or developmental quotients.

Cognitive Processes in the Learner,
and Customized MLE Components

In attempting to explain the neurological mechanisms of the psychological phenomenon of thinking, described as "an integral dynamic act" (p. 326), Luria (1973) delineates three major dynamic structural units of the central nervous system: arousal/attention, coding/analysis, and planning. These are now discussed in detail as they relate to the "customized" components of MLE.

Arousal/Attention

The first functional unit described by Luria is that of arousal/attention mechanisms, which maintain an optimal level of cortical tone, and thereby the waking state necessary for conscious mental activity. This tone or alertness is a by-product of the regulation of excitation and inhibition of brain activity, and can be behaviorally represented as "hyper-," "hypo-," or "optimal." When stimuli impinge upon the central nervous system, their acknowledgment and recognition are reflected in an "orienting response" — essentially, a momentary state of increased alertness in response to environmental change. Tone maintenance and regulation of excitation–inhibition following the initial orienting response comprise the mechanisms involved in attention. "Tone maintenance" describes the arousal function of the central nervous system, which relates to creation or maintenance of a state of alertness; "attention" refers to the more volitional aspects of directing focus to certain stimuli while ignoring others. (Since these functional systems are all interactive, no unit acts in isolation; therefore, it is important to note that both the coding and planning units [to be elaborated upon below] influence the attention/arousal mechanisms, and vice versa.)

In relation to educational tasks, Naglieri and Das (1989) comment that "during an attentional task, the child must work to direct activity and responsiveness to a particular stimulus and suppress reacting to a competing stimulus or stimuli" (p. 193); this is a description of "selective attention." In a later publication, Naglieri et al. (1990) distinguish between "focused attention" and "divided attention": "In focused attention the individual is required to attend to one kind of information and exclude others and in divided attention the individual shares time between two or more sources or kinds of information" (p. 427). Norman (1976) contributes to our understanding of attention the need to consider the match between the resources demanded by the task and the resources available within the child, thus introducing the issue of "attentional capacity" (e.g., span or "bits"). Tasks that have been mastered to the point of automaticity make little demand on attentional resources; tasks that are novel, complex, and demanding of processes not yet developed or mastered make much greater demands on attentional resources. In Norman's conceptualization, attention involves a voluntary directing of processing resources; this goes beyond a reactive model and is compatible with Luria's notion of the interaction of attentional, coding, and planning processes. This description also allows recognition of the idea that attention processes can be directed inward as well as outward, and enables us to account for the observation that some children appear unable to maintain attention to external stimuli (such as schoolwork) because of distraction by internal mental or physical stimuli. Thus, there is a differentiation between disturbances of the neurological mechanisms of attention (regulation) and disturbances that are interpretable as emotionally based because they involve distraction by anxiety-producing thoughts (it is assumed that these are not symptoms of psychosis).

Kirby and Grimley (1986) distinguish among "selective attention," "attentional capacity," and "sustained attention." Selective attention is "a person's ability to respond to the relevant aspects of a task or situation and to ignore or refrain from responding to irrelevant aspects"; attentional capacity is "the ability to attend to more than one stimulus at a time"; and sustained attention is the individual's ability to "maintain sensitivity to the requirements of a task and stay engaged in it over a period of time" (p. 12).

Kinsbourne and Caplan (1979) note, in discussing selective attention and attention capacity, that these reflect developmental level not only in terms of the number of elements to which the individual can attend at any one time, but in terms of the aspects of the stimulus that compel attention. For example, the features of form and color are likely to have greater attentional salience than features of size, location, orientation, or sequence (p. 56), especially for the young child. Even older children and adults may need to be taught to attend to the less salient features. Furthermore, what a child notes about the stimulus and how the stimulus situation is scanned greatly affects the mental processing that ensues, and thereby affects the act of thinking about the task or situation. Kinsbourne and Caplan support the dichotomy between auditory and visual attention; although the mechanisms of attention may be similar, the modality of expression may differ within and across children. For example, it is possible to conceive of a child who has attentional difficulty in the visual modality but not equal difficulty in the auditory, and vice versa.

What seems to develop regarding attentional processes is voluntary control; attention becomes increasingly guided by thinking (i.e., planning processes) (Vygotsky, 1986, p. 166). Day (cited in Fry & Lupart, 1987, p. 45) expands this further by delineating a number of aspects of attention that develop with age:

1. more systematic, task-appropriate strategies for acquiring visual information;
2. an increasing ability to maintain optimal performance across variations in the content and arrangement of stimuli;
3. visual scanning which becomes more exhaustive and more efficient;
4. an increasing focus on the portions of visual stimuli which are most informative for the specific task;
5. an increase in the speed of completion of visual search and comparison tasks;
6. an increase in the size of the useful "field of view."

Derived from the descriptions and definitions above, the attentional processes to be addressed in this model of dynamic assessment include the following:

1. Orienting response
2. Selective attention
3. Sustained attention
4. Divided attention

In addition to these processes, the assessor also notes the indicators of the child's attentional capacity, as well as the modality of attention expression (primarily visual or auditory, in the case of school-related work). Wittrock (1986, pp. 302–304) cites a number of research findings supporting the relationship between attentional processes and academic success.

The mediation offered by the assessor to address these processes includes those described in the "General Components" section as generally applicable, as well as the following. (The numbering here continues that of the earlier discussion.)

10. *Meaning*. Mediation of meaning helps to move the content from neutral to a position of value and importance. The mediator accomplishes this by affective emphasis — for example, through modulation of tone of voice, as well as by shows of enthusiasm. The mediator also articulates that certain content or elements are important and of value, and in this way contributes to the cultural socialization of the child. In addition, the mediator may highlight what is to be valued by inducing movement and by providing informational elaboration.

During the course of the assessment, the targeting of arousal and attention through mediation of meaning can take place when the assessor articulates to the child that it is important to pay attention and why (e.g., ". . . so you will know what to do"). The assessor also mediates meaning when tone of voice and affective expression are used to highlight aspects of the task to be selected for the child's focus. Comments such as "Wow, look at this! This is really pretty [unusual, weird, interesting, etc.]; do you see how it _____ ?" Mediation of meaning at its highest, or planning, level in relation to attentional processes may help the child understand how paying attention relates to the ability to gather complete information so that she will know what to do.

11. *Transcendence.* Mediation of transcendence involves promoting cognitive bridges between the task at hand and related but not currently present experiences of the child; these may refer to past experiences or those anticipated in the future. Transcendence at the highest level also promotes hypothetical and/or cause-and-effect reasoning. Mediation of transcendence helps to move the child from the perceptual to the conceptual, or from the concrete to the abstract. This component induces formulation of visual images, since the actual content is not present. Mediaton of transcendence is also a mechanism for promoting transfer of learning, since the child is helped to visualize situations that are not present, but that may be related to the current circumstances.

Targeting arousal and attention through mediation of transcendence may involve helping the child to think of other situations when it is important to pay attention (e.g., aspects of home or school that either facilitate or obstruct paying attention). For example, the assessor may ask, "Does this ever happen when you are with your group in school? Can we think of something to do when this happens?" This component can be used to promote transfer by discussing and role-playing or rehearsing situations related to the current involvement. For instance, the assessor can point out to the child how well it has worked to stand up every once in a while for doing work when feeling restless, and then talk about times during class when this might happen.

12. *Competence (task regulation).* Mediation of competence by means of task regulation refers to manipulation of the task to facilitate mastery by the child. Thus, the mediator provides verbal directions, intervenes nonverbally, or changes the task in ways that simplify or clarify it, in order to enable the child to succeed. Thus, task regulation accounts for a large proportion of the activities of teachers.

Targeting alertness and attention by mediation of task regulation occurs when the assessor paces presentation of materials to promote involvement, or provides types of materials (such as manipulables and other objects) that are colorful and attractive, or induces motor involvement. Most of all, mediation of task regulation at its highest level involves promoting the child's ability to succeed and providing feedback about what has and has not seemed to help him pay attention.

In addition to the above-described interventions that may be offered within the assessment situation, a number of approaches to promoting alertness and attention are available to teachers within the group instructional situation. These can be discussed with the teacher during feedback if it has been determined from the assessment that attention is an area in need of intervention. The assessor may then include these as recommendations in the assessment report, or as extensions of hypotheses from the assessment data.

Fry and Lupart (1987) offer the following generalizations, based on research for the facilitation of alertness within the classroom:

> Alertness is best maintained (1) when the task is varied, (2) feedback is provided, and (3) the learning situation is kept interesting to the students. . . . The optimal level of alertness, however, depends on the nature of the task. . . . Teachers need to recognize that short tasks built around concrete, personally relevant and meaningful problems keep the student[s] alert and active. (p. 47)

On the basis of these generalizations, Fry and Lupart recommend a number of specific strategies. To promote alertness, they suggest these tactics:

- Balanced variation of tasks (novelty, contrast, variety, surprise).
- Provision of feedback regarding how well students are doing.
- Keeping the situation interesting by use of "short tasks built around concrete, personally relevant and meaningful problems," as noted above.
- Arrangement of seating so that students who have difficulty with alertness are closer to the action.
- Regulation of the task difficulty so that the children can handle the demands.

To promote selective attention, Fry and Lupart suggest the following:

- Announcements of what is important and what needs to be noted; explicit statements of which features or elements to detect; awareness of what the children are likely to notice and what is likely to be overlooked; questions to promote processing of features to note (e.g., "Did you notice something about color that tells us which is the leaf and which is the flower?").
- Use of color and sound contrasts to highlight the features to note

(e.g., putting a red mark on the child's right hand to help teach right vs. left; saying the last word in a rhyme louder to emphasize the sameness of the endings; pointing to the item to be noticed).

• Elimination/reduction of irrelevant or distracting features (e.g., closing windows to reduce outside noise; covering items/pictures on a page not of immediate relevance; using earphones to enhance listening tasks, or study carrels to promote visual attention).

In addition, Wittrock (1986) suggests the following:

• Prequestions and articulation of lesson objectives to direct attention to specific elements.
• Postquestions to promote conceptualization regarding what preceded.
• Direct teaching of cognitive strategies such as self-talk ("How can I solve this? Am I following my plan? How did I do?").

Finally, Kirby and Grimley (1986) offer these suggestions:

• To reduce arousal, use of calming/relaxation procedures (e.g., muscle relaxation, breathing exercises).
• Breaking down tasks into component parts.

Coding/Analysis

The second functional unit of mental processing discussed by Luria (1966) is responsible for analysis and integration of information. This unit converts sensory stimuli into symbolic or concrete into abstract information; it includes the specific tasks of receiving and storing the information received from the senses (i.e., perception and memory, respectively). The types of coding processes discussed by Luria, "simultaneous" and "successive," are described as characterizing all of the subprocesses—that is, perception and memory, as well as the larger processing system of planning, and output mechanisms as well.

Although these coding processes may make neurological sense, it has been difficult to describe their educational relevance clearly. An attempt is made here to present the simultaneous and successive processes in as meaningful a way as possible. The two types of processing are discussed as they relate to the coding/analysis processes of perception and memory; they represent two ways in which information can be received and stored. These coding processes are relevant for the assessor to the extent that they are perceptible in working with the learner. Determination of the type of coding involved in a task may be relevant at the point of analysis of the task (i.e., what type of coding demands does the task make?), as well as in relation to how the child seems to be able to process the task demands; however, the degree to which analysis of coding in terms of simultaneous and successive processes can be meaningfully applied to the educational process remains to be determined.

Luria (1966) has described these two types of integrative processes, originally discussed by I. M. Sechenov in 1878, as follows:

> The first . . . is the integration of the individual stimuli arriving in the brain into simultaneous, and primarily spatial, groups, and the second is the integration of individual stimuli arriving consecutively in the brain into temporally organized, successive series [called, respectively] . . . simultaneous and successive synthesis. (p. 74)

The type of activity utilized appears to reflect the nature of the stimuli impinging upon the organism, with a match to the neurological capabilities required for processing. Examples of tasks involving simultaneous processing are copying geometric figures, construction of block designs, reading individual words, writing numerals, and grammatical structures involving spatial concepts (e.g., "Maria's father is my father's brother," or "Draw a circle above a square"). Examples of stimuli requiring successive processing include tapping out rhythms, imitating a series of movements, or repeating a series of numbers of unrelated words.

Especially in language, it can become quite confusing to determine whether successive or simultaneous processing is taking place, and it seems that these can overlap, depending upon the structure of the language (i.e., spatial or temporal). It also seems that individuals differ with regard to strategic preference for type of processing, so that the same input may be processed simultaneously or successively, depending upon the individual. Furthermore, as Vygotsky (1978) points out, what we perceive may be simultaneously integrated, but when we talk about it we are often restricted to the successive nature of speech (p. 33). Nevertheless, it may be possible to determine the type of coding process demanded by the particular task, as well as the type of coding process employed by the learner, and to determine whether there is a pattern that suggests a preference or facility with one type over the other.

Both simultaneous and successive processes are discussed in what follows to the extent that they relate to the specific processes. An attempt is also made to elaborate relevant educational implications.

Teaching strategies that attempt to reflect simultaneous versus successive (sequential) coding differences tend to emphasize analytic versus wholistic approaches. When applied to reading, for example, this translates into phonics versus "whole-word" methodology. Some success has been reported in facilitating achievement through an optimal match between the task's coding demands and the learner's coding preferences (e.g., Das, 1984; Kaufman & Kaufman, 1983); however, a number of unresolved issues and questions complicate investigation of the validity and interpretation of data regarding this essentially aptitude–treatment interaction (ATI) approach to education and remediation. Some of these issues include the following:

1. Not all learners can be clearly categorized in terms of these coding differences.

2. At times, the content presents a clear coding demand that is relatively independent of the learner's preference, and some content may be best learned by a method that is independent of learner preference. For example, if decoding is primarily sequential, and text organization and comprehension are primarily simultaneous, good readers need to have access to both modes of processing.

3. Some content may be processed by both types of coding or by varying combinations of the two; the specific coding demands are not always easily described or detected.

4. It continues to be debatable whether, to what extent, and in what cases weaknesses should be bypassed, strengthened, or compensated.

5. The theory is derived primarily from research on malfunctioning brains, and the application of its conclusions to normally developed neurological systems remains inferential.

Thus, it remains to be determined whether individuals can be meaningfully discriminated by coding preference, and, if so, whether this has significance for educational practice. For the purposes of the present assessment model, the two primary coding and integrative processes are presented as hypothetical descriptions of one aspect of mental activity. It may be useful for the assessor to be aware of the coding demands of the tasks presented and to be alert to the way they seem to be processed by the learner. The assessor can then try to determine whether patterns are discernible. If patterns are detected, and if these appear to be educationally meaningful, instructional connections can be hypothesized. One very frequently used example of how these differences in coding can be meaningful is to try to give driving directions to different people. Some "must" see the directions drawn, while others "need" to have them written out in narrative form; mismatches to coding preference or strength in this case may have very specific consequences.

In any event, one of the major strengths of dynamic assessment is that the assessment situation can be used as a laboratory to explore hypotheses for intervention. Assessors who perceive a pattern that seems to connect with a strength or a weakness can incorporate that perception into an on-the-spot trial intervention.

Perception Luria (1973) elaborates the receptive function of the brain in terms of "perception," defined as "an active process which includes the search for the most important elements of information, their comparison with each other, the creation of a hypothesis concerning the meaning of the information as a whole, and the verification of the hypothesis by comparing it with the original features of the object perceived" (p. 240). This describes what might be called a "search–detect–sort" process, where what is sought relates to what has been previously identified, sorted, and stored, and presumably functions in relation to affective need systems active at the time of perceptual activity (hypothesized in response to the need for a cause for the active search). Clearly, perception functions in relation to arousal and attention, and is influenced by the child's knowledge base and metacognitive capabilities. For the purpose of assessment, the aspects of behavior that are described as "perceptual" include the following:

1. Stimulus detection
2. Stimulus feature discrimination
3. Stimulus recognition
4. Stimulus comparisons
5. Perceptual strategies

The assessor must then respond to these questions:

1. Did the child detect (take note of the presence) of the stimulus? (If not, rule out sensory deficit.)

2. Was the child able to notice the distinctive features of the stimulus? (If not, rule out sensory deficit.)

3. Did the child attribute meaning to the stimulus? That is, was the child able to relate the stimulus to a previously stored label or percept?

4. Was the child able to engage in comparative operations either between two externally perceived percepts or between an externally perceived percept and stored information?

5. Did the child engage in any strategic behaviors—for example, regarding visual scanning?

In addition to the general mediational interventions described above, the assessor should address perceptual processes more specifically as follows.

Mediation of *meaning* that targets perceptual processes will help the child connect what is noted to his existing repertory of stored percepts and concepts. This may involve checking the child's knowledge base (e.g., does the child have a shape name vocabulary?), as well as memory storage and retrieval abilities. Elaboration of distinctive features and of their importance and value defines a high level of mediation of meaning.

Mediation of *task regulation* that addresses perceptual processes helps the child to make note of the distinctive features of an object or activity that will enable her to determine the degree and nature of sameness and difference. It may be necessary to increase the child's conceptual knowledge base by providing vocabulary to represent these features. At its highest level, mediation of task regulation helps the child to learn systematic scanning strategies with reference to a model, en route to facilitating the child's ability to compare. Provision and guidance of motor involvement with and exploration of objects may also enhance the child's awareness of distinctive features and the potential uses of the object; this also provides a means to reinforce application of strategic approaches (Fry & Lupart, 1987).

Mediation of *transcendence* that addresses perceptual processes will encourage the child to generalize strategies that have been learned to other related situations beyond the activity at hand. For example, in the case of strategic visual scanning, the mediator can ask the child: "Suppose all of a sudden I realize I dropped my keys on the playground; how could I go about finding them?" or "Are there other times we need to compare? Think about when we get dressed or go shopping for food. What do we compare at these times?"

Implications for the classroom teaching situation that relate to development of perceptual processes primarily involve attempts to increase the child's experiential knowledge base so that the child has repeated mediated exposure to the events and features to be perceived. The teacher needs to be explicit regarding the features to note, and should not assume that these features will have the same salience for a child as for an adult.

Teachers can also provide experiences that both highlight distinctive features and embed the features in their natural contexts (Norman, 1976, p. 61). For example, if children are to learn body parts, there should be opportunities to attend to the features of each part that make it special and identifiable, as well as to consider each part in relation to the whole body.

Fry and Lupart (1987) elaborate a number of classroom approaches to enhancing the perceptual functioning of children:

- For young children, encouragement of active visual and haptic exploration of the environment (young children seem to profit

more from self-guided exploration when initially introduced to a
new environment, whereas older children seem to profit more
from adult-guided exploration).

- Practice of discrimination training through use of cards that
provide comparison with a model, with mediation provided for
scanning strategies and information provided regarding what to
notice (sufficient exposure times must be provided, and complexity of features needs to be regulated).

Memory: Storage and Retrieval   Luria (1966) has described the
act of memorizing as "a complex process consisting of a series of
successive stages, differing in their psychological structure, in the
'volume' of traces capable of fixation, and in the duration of their
storage, and extending over a period of time" (p. 283). He specifies
three stages: first, imprinting of sensory cues (or, in the case of verbal
input, of phonetic features); second, transfer of the cues to image
memory; and, third, complex coding of traces and inclusion in a system
of categories (pp. 283–284). As he does for perception, Luria describes
memory as an active and dynamic process, requiring strategies to
convert short-term into long-term storage, as well as an optimal state of
arousal and vigilance.

Flavell (1985) offers some helpful definitions. Memory "in the wider
sense means the retention of all the products and achievements of one's
cognitive development to date" (p. 208). Storage and retrieval are
subcategories, defined as follows: "Storage activities put information
into memory while retrieval activities recover information from memory" (p. 208). Two frequently distinguished types of retrieval are
recognition and recall. "In recognition, the thing that is recognized is
already there to serve as its own retrieval cue. . . . In recall, the subject
has to do more of the retrieval job on his own" (p. 209). In infancy,
object permanence relates to the ability to recall, and is in evidence as
early as 9 months of age, if not earlier (Flavell, 1985, p. 212). Much of
what develops with increased age is the degree of intentionality
involved in storage and recall, as well as the increase in knowledge base.

There seems to be ongoing controversy regarding the types of
memory processes — specifically, whether there are different systems,
or whether apparent differences represent rates of decay within the
same system. A frequent distinction is made between short-term and
long-term memory. Specific strategies are described that facilitate the
transfer of short-term material into long-term storage. Furthermore,
there appears to be a neurological predisposition for organizing,
grouping, and clustering information into units that relate in terms of
subjective meaning (Norman, 1976). Memory is most often facilitated

by promoting meaningful associations between otherwise unrelated content (Wittrock, 1986), and by inducing active processing in the learner — that is, promoting mental processing that involves active manipulation of material to be recalled (e.g., moving it from one modality, such as verbal, into another, such as spatial). There thus appears to be an interaction between the promotion of meaningful connections and the active participation in this by the learner ("activity" implying mental manipulation).

The primary functions of the assessor and the teacher in relation to memory (specifically, storage and retrieval) processes are to facilitate the transfer of short-term into long-term memory, or storage, and to enhance the potential for retrieval. The assessor will wish to note whether the child has difficulty maintaining information in short-term memory, and, if so, to rule in or out the contribution of factors related to attention. The assessor should then try to note whether the child has any spontaneous strategies to promote storage and retrieval, and, if not, should offer those that appear relevant to the task and the child's level of functioning.

With this in mind, mediation of *meaning* that addresses memory involves explicit statements to the child that "this" is important to remember, and tries to attach an affective response to the content. The mediator also elaborates on characteristics of the object or experience that may generate interest in the child and that are highly differentiating of that object or experience. For example, if young children are given the opportunity to draw a picture, they can be given the choice of different implements to use, such as a pencil with an eraser, a pencil without an eraser, a crayon, or a marker; discussion can then ensue regarding the special features of each that relate to drawing (e.g., the presence vs. absence of an eraser, or the difference between a crayon and a pencil). The child's memory of the experience is likely to be enhanced by the experience of using each implement and exploring the possibilities of each.

Mediation of *transcendence* addressing memory processes includes promoting associations between the material to be learned and the child's previous experiences, as well as encouraging the child to convert material from one modality to another. For example, a frequently used mnemonic procedure is to promote the creation of visual imagery for verbal content (Wittrock, 1986). In the case of young children, this is best done by providing the pictorial images for them — for example, by drawing pictures to represent ideas, or by moving pictures around on a flannel board to act out a story being read (better yet, to have a child move the pictures in response to what he hears).

In another example, to teach the young child the concept of "circle," mediation can promote the association between a circle and a ball.

During initial phases of learning, the words may be repeatedly paired —
for example, referring to the shape as "circle ball." In this way, retrieval
is enhanced by being able to give one of the pair as a cue for eliciting
the second member of the pair (Wittrock, 1986).

The mediator should encourage the child to generate her own
connections, after many such examples have been provided; however,
it is important to be aware that such spontaneous generation of
connections is difficult if not impossible for some young children
(Weinstein & Mayer, 1986), and they should not be unduly frustrated
by such attempts.

Mediation of *task regulation* that addresses memory processes includes
use of the great variety of learning strategies available to promote
metacognitive development, and to help the child to apply metacognitive capacities to learning demands. These may include helping the
child to think of ways to organize or "chunk" material to promote
retention, and to model and practice the use of rehearsal strategies
(Norman, 1969; Weinstein & Mayer, 1986). At the preschool level,
early rehearsal strategies include encouraging the child to name, point
to, and manipulate the content to be retained (Fry & Lupart, 1987, p.
105).

It should be clear that the child's memory is strongly related to his
knowledge base — that is, to information previously encoded and
stored. Children with a broader and more extensive experience base
may be expected to have more potential sources for promoting
connections. It is therefore important for children to develop an
age-appropriate experience base in order to develop optimal learning
potential, under the assumption that learning and memory are inextri-
cably interconnected.

In applying thinking about mediation of memory to the classroom,
both Weinstein and Mayer (1986) and Fry and Lupart (1987) provide
recommendations of potential usefulness for teachers. Weinstein and
Mayer (1986, pp. 316–317) list and discuss eight major categories of
learning strategies that apply to students of varying ages (not all
strategies apply to all ages):

1. Rehearsal strategies for basic learning styles (e.g., "repeating the
   names of items").
2. Rehearsal strategies for complex learning tasks (e.g., "copying,
   underlining, shadowing material").
3. Elaboration strategies for basic learning tasks (e.g., "forming a
   mental image or sentence relating the items").
4. Elaboration strategies for complex tasks (e.g., "paraphrasing,
   summarizing, or describing how new information relates to
   existing knowledge").

5. Organizational strategies for basic learning tasks (e.g., "grouping or ordering to-be-learned items").
6. Organizational strategies for complex tasks (e.g., "outlining a passage or creating a hierarchy").
7. Comprehension-monitoring strategies (e.g., "checking for comprehension failures [via] . . . self-questioning").
8. Affective strategies (e.g., "being alert and relaxed, to help overcome test anxiety").

In general, the strategies above that involve complex learning tasks are not applicable to young children (i.e., children younger than 11 to 12 years). Also, even in the case of basic learning tasks, it is necessary when the learner is below age 8 for the mediator to be explicit and to offer concrete examples of the strategies, rather than expecting the child to produce them spontaneously.

Fry and Lupart (1987) offer a number of suggestions that are particularly relevant for working with young children. These include the following:

1. Emphasis on visual/iconic (picture) processing.

2. Encouragement of recoding material from one modality into another (e.g., visual/iconic to echoic/auditory). For example, this might include following a presentation of a lesson presented on a TV screen with a brief discussion of the content.

3. Early encouragement of rehearsal by means of naming, pointing, and manipulation of materials.

4. Presentation of material in preorganized chunks. For example, when a teacher is trying to help children remember their phone number, it is likely that they will remember 529-4697 better than 5294697 (a phenomenon most adults have learned well).

5. Promotion of storing information in categories (e.g., colors, numbers, shapes, etc.) This is often done in preschool programs in terms of presentation of material as units. That is, the teacher rarely says, "Today we are going to talk about police, fireworkers, medical people, and food preparers"; more often than not, the teacher introduces this material in terms of a unit on community helpers.

6. Provision of directions with awareness of the effects of primacy and recency. That is, children will be likely to remember the last thing that they hear; therefore, the most important thing to remember should be said last (this also implies that instructions should be kept short).

7. Provision of information that takes note of high-salience and high-specificity effects. That is, the characteristics of an object or task that are special and specific to that object or task, and that are likely to hold a high degree of salience for a child of a certain age, should be

emphasized. For example, in discussing animals in the zoo, it is more likely that the child will remember that a zebra has stripes than that the zebra is shorter and thicker than a horse.

8. Clear statements of the intent and goal of remembering. The children need to be told explicitly to listen in order to remember, or to try to remember, because they will be asked questions afterward.

Planning

Although planning processes have been built into each of the areas described above as the optimal expression and objective of mediation, further discussion is warranted because this is a functional unit discussed specifically by Luria and aligned with identifiable neurological correlates. Luria sees the capacity for planning as enabling the most human of functions. It is the capacity for planning to which he attributes the active role of individuals in their experiences. According to Luria, a person "creates intentions, forms plans and programmes of his actions, inspects their performance, and regulates his behavior so that it conforms to these plans and programmes; finally, he verifies his conscious activity, comparing the effects of his actions with the original intentions and correcting any mistakes he has made" (1966, p. 80). Thus Luria describes the executive or metacognitive capacity of the human. Planning interacts with arousal and attention through self-regulation and impulse control, and planning interacts with coding processes through selection and adjustment of strategies. The assessor interacting with the learner needs to observe and test out how effectively the child utilizes self-regulatory processes, and how well developed the coding strategies are. The assessor, as mediator, should work toward inducing planning in the child.

Finally, putting all the pieces together into the mental activity called "thinking," Luria has proposed:

> Thinking arises only when the subject has an appropriate motive which makes the task urgent and its solution essential, and when the subject is confronted by a *situation for which he has no ready-made (inborn or habitual)* solution. . . . The next stage [is] . . . the *restraining* of impulsive responses, the *investigation of the conditions* of the problem, the analysis of its components, recognition of the most essential features, and their correlation with one another. . . . The third stage . . . is the *selection of one from a number of possible alternatives* and the creation of a *general plan (scheme) for the performance* of the task . . . [that is,] the general *strategy*. . . . The next (fourth) phase of thinking . . . is choosing the appropriate *methods* and considering which *operations* will be adequate for putting the general scheme of the solution into effect. . . . (1966, pp. 327–328; italics in original)

Thus, within this conceptualizaton, thinking cannot take place without a feeling of dissonance or discrepancy — a need to regain equilibrium or balance, or possibly to move ahead to new territory. When the child does not recognize or admit to this basic motivating need, it is up to the mediator to try to provoke or help the child to recognize such a discrepancy as the primary motivation for problem solving, and therefore for thinking. Once motivated, the mediator then works to facilitate development of the most optimal problem-solving approaches — approaches that are internalized by the child and available for independent application to situations when the mediator is no longer present.

A Tabular Representation of the Model

Now that the reader has been introduced to the components of this basic model of preschool dynamic assessment, it may be helpful to present all of the assessment components in tabular form. The assessment model attempts to account for the three primary interactive components of the assessment situation: the task, the learner, and the assessor. Task components of content, processes tapped, operations required, modalities involved, and levels of abstraction, complexity, and efficiency have been introduced (see Appendix III.B). Learner processes of arousal/attention, coding, and planning, as well as the learner's knowledge base, have been described. Finally, the mediational components of intentionality, meaning, transcendence, sharing (shared focus and sharing of experience), competence (praise/encouragement, challenge, and task regulation), psychological differentiation, change, contingent responsivity, and affective involvement have been elaborated.

The task components provide implications for potential for transfer, in that the results of the assessment may be expected to apply to situations that share components with the task incorporated into the assessment. The learner processes have implications for conclusions about the learner's modifiability and for profiling of the learner's cognitive strengths and weaknesses. Finally, the mediational components have implications for observations of the types of input that promote changes in the learner, the intensity required for such change, and for hypotheses for interventions that show promise of successful promotion of learning. These can be portrayed as shown in Table III.1.

The general dynamic assessment model has now been fully presented. What remains is to describe the expression of this general model in two specific applications: a "generic" version that specifically targets

TABLE III.1. Model for Preschool Dynamic Assessment

Task components	Learner processes	Mediational components
Content	Knowledge base	Intentionality
Processes	Arousal/attention	Meaning
Operations	Coding	Transcendence
Complexity	Perception	Sharing
Abstraction	Memory	Shared focus
Efficiency	Planning	Sharing of experience
Modalities	Output	Psychological differentiation
		Contingent responsivity
		Competence
		Praise/encouragement
		Challenge
		Task regulation
		Affective involvement
		Change
	Implications for:	
Transfer	Modifiability	Nature and intensity
	Strengths/weaknesses	of input
		Interventions

preschool children, and a curriculum-based adaptation applicable primarily to preschoolers, but usable with older (school-age) children as well.

THE PRESCHOOL LEARNING ASSESSMENT DEVICE: A "GENERIC" APPROACH

Introduction

The Preschool Learning Assessment Device (PLAD) utilizes a group of typical preschool "readiness" tasks to gain insight into the learning abilities of children from the ages of 3 through 5. There is a general test–intervene–retest format; three tasks, with process demands related to the pretest and posttest, comprise the intervention portion. Each of these intervention tasks is presented in a test–intervene–retest format as well, which yields a total of four opportunities for the assessor to assess change in the learner on each task. The entire procedure is anchored to the Triangles subtest of the Kaufman Assessment Battery for Children (K-ABC; Kaufman & Kaufman, 1983), selected because it is a frequently used psychometric procedure, likely to be incorporated into a preschool assessor's battery. This permits a connection of the dynamic with the psychometric procedure, so that some picture of the child is derived of functioning in terms of both a static and a dynamic format.

The intervention tasks include human (child) figure drawing, building steps with 10 cubes, and copying parquetry designs. The materials required are as follows: the Triangles subtest from the K-ABC, paper and pencil for the figure drawing, 20 one-color 1-inch cubes for the steps, and the large wooden block parquetry set from Developmental Learning Materials (see address in the "Resources" section of this book). It is also helpful to have a puzzle-like human figure for the intervention phase of the figure drawing.

The (subjective) task analysis of the activities is portrayed in Table III.2. As can be seen in the table, there is considerable overlap among the activities in the processes, operations, modalities, levels of complexity, and efficiency (in terms of speed) involved. There is more variety and divergence with regard to content, level of abstraction, and efficiency (in terms of precision). These parameters define the characteristics of tasks to which the results of this assessment may be generalized.

The overall model of administration is as follows:

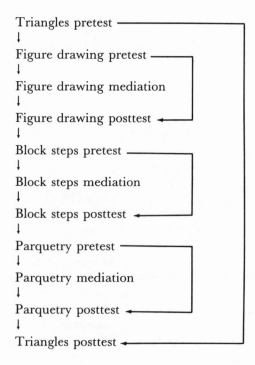

Triangles pretest

Figure drawing pretest

Figure drawing mediation

Figure drawing posttest

Block steps pretest

Block steps mediation

Block steps posttest

Parquetry pretest

Parquetry mediation

Parquetry posttest

Triangles posttest

TABLE III.2. Analysis of PLAD Tasks

			Tasks	
Aspect	Triangles	Figure drawing	Block steps	Parquetry
Content	Plastic triangles, each yellow on one side/blue on other; stimulus pictures	Paper, pencil, puzzle figure	20 one-color, 1-inch cubes; blank paper	Multicolored parquetry pieces; blank paper; stimulus pictures (rocket design)
Processes	Attention (selective and sustained); simultaneous coding; perceptual analysis; retrieval of shape and color concepts; planning strategies	Same	Same	Same
Operations	Matching, comparing, discriminating, sensory–motor integration, part–whole analysis	Sensory–motor integration, comparing, part–whole analysis	Comparing, part–whole analysis, sensory–motor integration	Sensory–motor integration, comparing, discriminating, part–whole analysis
Modalities	Visual, tactile, kinesthetic, spatial	Visual, pictorial, graphic, spatial	Visual, tactile, kinesthetic, spatial	Visual, tactile, kinesthetic, pictorial, spatial
Complexity[a]	4	4	3	4
Abstraction[a]	5	1	2	3
Efficiency[a]				
Speed	2	2	2	2
Precision	4	3	5	5

[a]These aspects are rated on a scale of 1 to 5, and represent my estimates.

151

This list not only shows the order of administration of the tasks, but demonstrates the possibility of deriving four change scores or observations as a result of this procedure. All activities in these procedures are introduced to the child in a problem-solving-inducing format. Thus, when materials are placed in front of the child, the directions are not quickly offered. The child is first asked, "Do you know what these are? What do you think I will ask you to do with these?" This type of presentation is important to maintain, because the child is informed by this that she is expected to be an active processer in this interaction. This procedure also differs from traditional approaches in the assessor's degree of explicitness in discussing what is observed and what is going on throughout the course of the assessment. The assessor informs the child of the objectives of the assessment — that is, what problems have been observed and what will be addressed — and continues to articulate what seems to work or not to work, encouraging the child's observations and input at all times. Except during the pretest phases (which are administered in traditional static format), the assessor provides elaborated feedback to the child regarding the correctness of responses, and, most of all, elaborations regarding what seems to help or obstruct the achievement of success. In other words, the assessor provides optimal mediation in terms of the components discussed above.

For most preschool children, the PLAD should require about 1 to $1\frac{1}{2}$ hours. It is likely that some breaks (bathroom, drinks, snacks, walks) will be necessary. The pretests can be separated from the rest of the procedure, but it is particularly important that the intervention and posttests be completed during the course of one assessment session. The PLAD is best administered as the last of several assessment procedures. Prior to the procedure, the assessor should have analyzed the processing needs of the child; further information regarding processes in need of intervention should be gleaned from the pretests within the PLAD. The entire procedure is introduced to the child with comments such as the following: "We are now going to do some teaching and learning together. I noticed in our work that you seemed to have some difficulty with _____ . We can work on this today to see whether we can find some ways to help you to be a better learner."

Administration Procedures

1. Administration of the Triangles subtest of the K-ABC according to standardized instructions. (If this has already been administered as part of the assessment battery, these results can be used.)

2. Administration of the figure drawing pretest. The assessor should

present the child with a blank sheet of paper turned vertically, with a primary-size pencil, and ask the child first what he thinks he will be doing. (Alternatively, the assessor can tell the child that they will next be drawing, and then can present only the paper or the pencil and ask the child, "Do you have everything you need? Can you go ahead with your drawing?"). The child is then asked to "draw a picture of a child — a boy or a girl."

3. Mediation of figure drawing. This is customized in accord with the perceived needs of the child; however, one possible intervention is work involving reference to a human figure puzzle, with the opportunity to play a game of missing or dislocated parts that includes giving the child the chance of playing "teacher" and hiding or misplacing parts while the assessor closes her eyes. Another recommended intervention is to remove the drawing implement from the child, and ask the child to play "teacher" and tell the assessor how to draw the picture. The child may need very explicit guidance through this. For example: "What shall we draw, a boy or a girl? Where shall we start, with the head or with the feet? Where do the [feet] go? What shape shall we use?" and so forth.

4. Administration of the figure drawing posttest, with the same instructions as the pretest.

5. Mediation of change; the assessor and child compare the pretest and posttest.

6. Administration of the block steps pretest. The assessor should place 10 blocks in front of the child and ask, "Do you know what these are? What can we do with them?" The child is then told that the assessor will build something with them, but will hide it behind a paper screen so that the child cannot see the blocks until the entire configuration is complete. When the final product is ready, the child is asked to look carefully at it: "Do you think you can build one like that?" The assessor then takes down the product and asks the child to "build one just like mine," offering that "if it is hard for you, we will work on it just the way that we worked on the drawing." The child's production is recorded in a sketch.

7. Mediation of the block steps task. This can include provision of a model and discussion of different ways to proceed, emphasizing part–whole analysis to the child. The assessor can point out to the child that the construct can be made either with "trains" or with "towers" (i.e., horizontal rows or vertical stacks), and the child can be given the choice of which one to try. The assessor should also mediate meaning by inducing a label from the child and emphasizing the need to leave one block sticking out so that there is room for the foot to step on it.

8. Administration of the block steps posttest, when the child seems to have had sufficient mediation; the same instructions are given as in the pretest, and the final production is sketched out.

9. Mediation of change between pretest and posttest.

10. Administration of the pretest of the parquetry designs. The design used for pre- and posttesting is a rocket-like drawing. The blocks needed to reproduce the picture are preselected for the child. The model picture is placed above a similarly oriented blank sheet of paper, and the child is again asked to think of what needs to be done here. The assessor then tells the child to "make a picture just like this one" on the blank sheet, again offering that if it seems very hard, "we will learn to do it just like we did the drawing and the steps." A quick sketch is made of the child's final product. (Alternatively, a Polaroid photograph can be used.)

11. Mediation using one of two pictures with related configurations; the child is asked which one she prefers to learn on. The child is first allowed to place the blocks directly on the design. Next, the child is asked to make the picture on a separate piece of paper that has the lines of the figure drawn in. Finally, the child is asked to make the figure on a blank sheet of paper. The specifics of the mediation need to address the difficulties that the child seems to be experiencing.

12. Posttest with the same rocket design; the child's results are sketched.

13. Mediation of change.

14. Readministration of the K-ABC Triangles subtest.

During the course of this procedure, the assessor needs to be making notes describing the processing needs of the child, as well as recording the types of interventions that seem to help or not to help. It is also important to note any signs of spontaneous applications of what has been learned during the course of the interaction, as well as original contributions of the child.

Assessors need to be cautioned not to mediate on the pretest and posttest, because these are used to derive an objective indication of a child's ability to change and to function without an assessor's guidance. Assessors specifically need to be reminded not to provide labels for a child during the pretests — for example, for the steps or for the rocket — as derivation of meaning and retrieval of a relevant percept will become part of the mediational process. Although the procedure may appear complex at first, it is important for assessors not to fear making mistakes. Such struggles can become part of the "sharing" process, and can be explicitly articulated for the child as part of the mediation. It is also helpful during occasional necessary delays to engage in self-talk, so that the child is kept informed about what is going on, and even the delays can become part of the learning process. For example, the child can be informed that new materials are being prepared; that it will take a few seconds to pick out the blocks so that the child can have all that he needs; and that the assessor needs just a few minutes to write out some notes, so that all the work that is being done together can be remembered at a later time. The initial recording of results as the assessment is taking place is done with the form in Appendix III.A. These "raw" results are then used to complete the "Summary of Dynamic Assessment Results" presented in Appendix III.C. The information from this summary report can be utilized directly, or can be incorporated into a larger, more comprehensive report. If relevant, the information can also be drafted into Individualized Educational Program (IEP) format as outlined in Appendix III.D. The checklist in Appendix III.E can serve to guide assessors through the necessary steps.

A CURRICULUM-BASED DYNAMIC ASSESSMENT APPROACH

The flexibility of dynamic assessment allows adapting it to a curriculum-based approach, as well as the "generic" approach offered by the PLAD, which incorporates predetermined tasks appropriate to a specific age level. A curriculum-based version of dynamic assessment differs from diagnostic teaching in the continued focus on cognitive processing (albeit, in this case, as applied to curriculum content). The test–intervene–retest format still applies, as does the mediational approach to the intervention phase. What differs is that the specific tasks selected for content and for pre- and posttesting are taken directly from the child's curriculum, and should reflect content with which the child is demonstrating learning difficulty.

The steps of the curriculum-based dynamic assessment procedure are as follows:

1. Selection of a task from the curriculum with which the child is experiencing difficulty. The assessor should develop three versions of this task, all of which should be at an equal level of difficulty.

2. Review of the cognitive process list (in Appendix III.A), with an eye to the processes that appear relevant to the task; also, analysis of the task in accord with Appendix III.B.

3. Administration of the first form of the task as a 5- to 10-minute pretest. The assessor should not intervene; he should merely record the child's responses, and make notations regarding the difficulties the child seems to experience in terms of the process list (and any previous

knowledge the assessor may have of the child's functioning on these types of tasks).

4. Mediation, using the second form of the same task. The mediation should reflect the MLE components described earlier in this manual, as well as educational practices known to be best for the type of activity involved. Prior to the mediation, the assessor should think through some possible interventions. Here are some additional aspects to consider:

a. Is the task at an appropriate level for this child (not too easy or too difficult)?
b. Do the the language/concept demands of the task and of instructions need to be modified?
c. What should be done to promote the attention of the child?
d. How should the task be regulated for this child?
e. How can the child be helped to remember what was learned?
f. How can the child be helped to transfer what was learned to other situations?

5. Recording of notes during the course of the mediation to indicate what is being worked on, what the child's needs seem to be, how the child is responding, what seems to work and seems not to work, and so on.

6. Posttesting, using the third version of the task. Again, the assessor should not intervene, but just record the child's responses.

7. Mediation of change to the child, comparing pre- and postintervention performances, with elaborations regarding what has changed.

8. Completion of the assessment summary sheet (Appendix III.C), and of an IEP if relevant (Appendix III.D).

9. Development of a lesson based on the results of the assessment (Appendix III.F).

10. Scheduling and evaluation of teaching sessions based on the results of the assessment (Appendix III.G).

The curriculum-based approach to dynamic assessment is relevant for teachers and educational diagnosticians, but also allows other assessors to address curriculum content quite directly. This model thus provides the ultimate link to classroom instruction, since it incorporates both instructional strategies and instructional content. The list of competencies listed in Appendix III.H should allow assessors to check their own skills, as well as to facilitate training of other assessors within this approach.

If the referral of the child describes difficulty with mastering curriculum objectives, and if the assessor has direct access to a specific curriculum, it becomes relevant to carry out this curriculum-based procedure. When the concerns about the learner's response to instruction are more diffuse and/or the child is not in an educational program, and/or the assessor can not easily access the child's curriculum content, it becomes more relevant to carry out a more generic type of dynamic assessment (e.g., the PLAD).

RESEARCH

The research available to date that specifically includes the PLAD, or the model of dynamic assessment on which it is based, is very limited. The model and the procedure are presented here in great detail with the hope of encouraging further investigation. The research on dynamic assessment as elaborated in other models and as a general concept is reviewed in Chapter 5 of Part I. The two studies that have been carried out so far using the PLAD are reviewed here.

I have collaborated with two students whose doctoral dissertations included work with the PLAD, as first elaborated elsewhere (Lidz & Thomas, 1987). The first study was conducted by Thomas (1986). The subjects were 60 Head Start children, mostly black and Hispanic, between the ages of 3 and 5 years, who had been referred for assessment because of teachers' concerns about their difficulty learning in or adjusting to their programs. The study focused on the effects of the mediation offered during the administration of the PLAD procedure; the experimental group received mediation, and the control group had unmediated experience with the same materials for the same amount of time, in the presence of the assessor. The study also looked at the relationship between the performance of the children in the mediated and unmediated groups and their scores on the California Preschool Competency Scale for Children, completed by their teachers. The mediated children made significant gains on their posttest scores, whereas the unmediated group showed virtually no change in their performance in the posttesting. Significant and strong correlations were found between the magnitude of the gains and the scores on the social competency measure.

The second study (Reinharth, 1989) included 36 developmentally delayed children between the chronological ages of 2 years, 7 months and 11 years, with mental ages between 20 and 63 months; experimental and control groups were matched on a number of variables, including age and cognitive level. This group included children of mixed socioeconomic levels (ranging between low and upper-middle income groups), but was predominantly white. Like the Thomas (1986) study, this study focused on the effects of mediation between experimental and control groups; again, the controls were offered exposure to the materials without mediation. The results were also similar in that there were highly significant differences in pre- and posttest scores for the mediated group, but not for the controls. A unique aspect of this study was a retest of performance 2 weeks after the posttest. The intent was to check stability of effects. What Reinharth found was an increase in the differences between groups, with the mediated group further increasing their posttest gains, and the controls remaining the same with no changes.

Although there are some technical difficulties with these studies, such as use of gain scores and use of the same assessor for pre- and posttesting as well as mediation, the results of both are strong and reinforcing of each other, despite the differences in populations and differences in assessors across studies. Obviously, more work is needed.

What follows are case reports of three children with whom dynamic assessment approaches, usually incorporating the PLAD, have been used. These will provide the reader with examples of the type of information generated by this model, as well as samples of integration of this information with prescriptive recommendations.

SAMPLE PSYCHOEDUCATIONAL ASSESSMENT REPORTS

Case 1

Name: Ronald Doe

Chronological Age: 5 years, 9 months

Reason for Referral: Mrs. and Mrs. Doe have requested assessment of their son, Ronald, by means of a dynamic assessment model in order to gain some insight into his learning capabilities, and to contribute to their planning for his educational future. They specifically do not wish for standardized testing, as they do not feel that this type of information is meaningful in their son's case.

Background Information: Ronald has been evaluated over the years by a number of professionals. These records are available from the early intervention center and are in his current program file. Ronald's current educational classification is "neurologically impaired," and his condition has been diagnosed by a neurologist as "static encephalopathy that was manifested by central hypotonia." The neurologist's most current (1989) evaluation notes significant improvement "in all areas of function, including his socialization, his muscular hypotonia, and above all his expressive language."

Ronald is currently in an integrated program in his early intervention center; that is, his classroom includes children with and without developmental delays. He also is involved in occupational and physical therapy, as well as swimming and dancing programs at the YMCA. He has had eye surgery to correct a condition resulting in double vision, and has an astigmatism. He is being considered for glasses. He had both feet in casts, but these casts were recently removed. His mother describes him as very affectionate and eager to please; he presents no behavior problems, and his parents take him everywhere.

Ronald's current teacher notes his increased awareness, and finds that he is often more aware than he appears. He can seem to be tuned out, but is then able to respond accurately to a question just discussed. He is also improved in his ability to respond to group directions. She finds that he needs attention to expanding his interactions, staying on task, and acquiring classroom routines. He has mastered many basic concepts, is able to read letters and numbers, and can count to 10 with one-to-one correspondence. He responds best to a very enthusiastic response, and needs his work presented very systematically, with modeling and practice. Lessons need to be game-like. His social interaction is estimated at a 3- to 4-year-old level. He is left-hand-dominant, and his fine motor limitations are evident in class, affecting his acquisition of writing skills. He has difficulty with finger differentiation and with effecting a pincer grasp. Continuation of occupational therapy will probably be needed.

Ronald's speech therapist reports good progress as well. He is working on "wh-" questions, following directions, and classifying objects. He shows incidental learning and good spontaneous language. The therapist has found it helpful to ring a bell when he gets something correct. She also sees him as more spontaneous and more able to "catch on" than other special needs children in the program. He will need to continue his speech/language therapy on at least a twice-a-week basis.

Procedures:

- File review
- Classroom observation
- Parent interview
- Teacher interview
- Speech/language pathologist interview
- Observation and interaction with Ronald, with informal use of the

Goodman Lock Box, the Triangles subtest from the Kaufman Assessment Battery for Children (K-ABC), and human figure drawing

Assessment Results: This is neither a comprehensive nor a standardized psychoeducational assessment. This is a descriptive report based on informal measures in order to provide insight into Ronald's current functioning and future educational needs.

Within his classroom, Ronald is manageable and compliant. He responds appropriately to routines and participates both verbally and nonverbally in group activities. He appears happy, and relates well to the adults in the program; he delights in praise and encouragement. In a free-play situation with peers, however, he tends to keep to himself and does not spontaneously interact with the other children. While ambulating, he is awkward (the awkwardness may be exacerbated by the recent removal of his casts), and does not use his eyes well to direct his gross motor movements. He also shows difficulty with spatial judgment — for example, trying to seat himself in a toy highchair, and bumping a vehicle he is pushing into objects in his path.

In individual sessions, Ronald is pleasant and relates well. He begins most tasks willingly, but is easily and quickly frustrated by challenge. A major obstruction to his success is his difficulty with fine motor skills. He has a history of hypotonicity, which, although reportedly improved, seems to have laid the groundwork for anticipated failure and frustration. Since so many tasks for young children include a perceptual-motor component, Ronald has a history of being constantly exposed to materials that present challenges to him but that would not be challenging for another child of his age without his motor limitations. He also seems to have a temperamental predisposition to withdraw from rather than persist with confrontations to his ability.

Adults working with Ronald have found it effective to maximize his success experiences; to embed new learning in the security of already mastered material; and to reinforce learning with large doses of praise, encouragement, and occasional concrete reinforcement (hugs and kisses usually suffice). Use of a timer to signal the end of a work or play period has also been more successful than merely telling him to stop; however, use of such devices is rarely necessary, and needs to be considered an alternative only when other approaches are not successful.

Ronald's most dramatic gain during the past year has been in his development of language. He is able to use language to express his needs and desires, and to manipulate his world in order to get his needs met. At this time, his use of language is fairly routinized and at a concrete level, although he can use language to label emotions, and is capable of inferring verbal opposites. At this time, he is limited in his inferential ability and his use of language for problem solving. He is also more proficient in his communication with adults than with peers.

The combination of major changes in Ronald's development during the past year and his continuing delays in both motor and language domains, complicated by his limited attention span and persistence, makes it impossible to estimate his capacities with any accuracy. That is, he is very much in the process of major change. At the same time, access to his ability to learn is still hampered by the nature of his limitations.

Working with Ronald within a dynamic assessment format has demonstrated his ability to respond positively even to short-term interventions, while also illustrating his difficulties with persistence and attention maintenance. It was possible to observe Ronald's performance with two tasks using this format: the Triangles subtest from the K-ABC, and a human figure drawing task. It was possible to carry out the Triangles subtest only in an interventionist format, without clear pre- and posttests, but Ronald's response to the intervention was nevertheless dramatic. He progressed from being unable to deal with the task to independent solution of items (at his age, only one or two independent successes would place him within "normal" range). What seemed to help was to provide him with a "strategy routine." The assessor showed him how to create a large triangle with two smaller triangles by noting the length of the sides and by verbalizing a "short–short–long" rhythm routine. Ronald quickly absorbed this "short–short–long" strategy and used it spontaneously via self-talk to guide his solution of the items. As the assessor withdrew her attention to write some notes, Ronald proceeded to solve the next item successfully without intervention. What did not seem to work with him — a finding that corroborates his continuing language and symbolic delays — was an attempt to enhance the meaning of the triangles by giving them real-life labels (e.g., "Mommy" and "Daddy"). This type of intervention served more to muddy than to clarify his understanding.

Similarly dramatic was Ronald's response to the human figure drawing task, which was administered in test–intervene–retest format. First of all, his parents had been informed from a previous attempt to evaluate him that he was not able to draw a human figure. However, during this assessment, even without intervention, Ronald was clearly able to produce a recognizable figure with a head and scribbled arms and feet. This attests to the difficulty with drawing conclusions about Ronald's abilities from one single attempt to assess him. Furthermore, despite his fine motor difficulty and his attitudinal resistance to engaging in further "work," Ronald showed responsiveness to the intervention by producing a much more articulated, controlled figure. He also showed improved spatial positioning of the arms and legs of the puzzle figure used during the intervention phase. What seemed to help in this task were, first, references to his own body; and, second, having him "teach" the assessor what to do by telling her what part to draw and where to put it, and observing the model produced for him from this. In this case, removing the motor aspect of the task (the assessor drew; he talked) and forcing him to "think" seemed to help when it was again his turn to draw.

Ronald's response to the Goodman Lock Box, a structured play assessment procedure, showed the degree to which his ability to show his capacity is obstructed by his fine motor limitations and his avoidant response to this type of task demand. He was clearly curious about the contents lying behind the locked doors, but would attempt only the easiest locks, and would only try to peer through the cracks of the closed doors without being able to overcome his inhibitions. When he was left to his own devices and intervention was withheld, he retreated to self-stimulatory behavior. Adult intervention is clearly needed to help him overcome his tendency to retreat when faced with this type of obstacle, and to maintain his external engagement.

Ronald's mastery of some academic content (counting, colors, letters) attests to his responsiveness to teaching and to his adequate memory processes, once his attention is focused. He also demonstrates good ability to do sequential tasks involving pattern detection, and is able to complete verbal opposites on his computer programs. His attention is held very successfully by these computer programs.

Analysis of the pretest–posttest results accomplished by Ronald's current program show that he has made gains in the vicinity of 15 to 18 months over a 9-month period of time. His performance levels are uneven across domains, with strengths in tasks involving visual perception and, in some cases, comprehension. His weaknesses in the fine motor area and in attention maintenance are evident. It is also relevant to note that there is some inconsistency across tests, with different levels of performance indicated by different tests. This may reflect limitations of the tests themselves, but may also reflect fluctuations in Ronald's attentiveness at the time of testing. When he is focused, he can perform at a relatively high level; when he is unfocused, he is "gone," and gives random responses without cognitive investment.

Although this assessment has not produced scorable results and does not provide enlightenment regarding Ronald's levels of performance, on the one hand there is evidence that Ronald is capable of working on some tasks that are within expectations for his chronological age; on the other hand, it also demonstrates that Ronald's level of performance varies in response to how he is handled and to what extent he is "tuned in." These results do show that he is a capable responder to intervention.

Recommendations:

1. Ronald is currently classified as "neurologically impaired." This continues to appear to be the most appropriate educational classification. Placement in a small classroom appropriate for children so classified is supported. Ronald needs ready access to his teachers, who need to be available to provide ongoing encouragement and reinforcement.

2. Ronald would profit from increased demands on his problem-solving skills. This can be accomplished in a variety of ways. For example, adults can "talk aloud" their own problem solving as a model for him. They can also interact with him in a question-asking way:

- What do you need to do?
- What's the problem here?
- What's missing?
- What should we do first?
- What can we do about this?
- If we do _____ , what will happen?

To promote his ability to respond to these questions, it may be necessary (a) to ask the question rhetorically (i.e., ask and then answer), and encourage his imitation; and (b) to ask a peer to respond and then encourage his imitation.

3. Ronald's social interaction may be promoted by reduced direct instruction, but increased provision of sideline coaching plus encouragement of more socially developed peers to initiate interactions with him.

4. Ronald's learning seems to be enhanced by providing him with verbal routines, which he can then repeat as self-talk. For new learning, it is suggested that the solutions be verbalized aloud by the adult in the form of short rhythms, similar to the "short–short–long" routine of the Triangles test.

5. Ronald's parents have expressed interest in the Cognitive Education Curriculum for Young Children developed at the Kennedy Center of Vanderbilt University. The assessor will provide information regarding its imminent publication.

6. Consultation with Ronald's occupational therapist is recommended to explore positioning alternatives that may enhance his ability to attend to tasks.

7. Overcoming Ronald's resistance to challenge and increasing his task persistence need to be very explicit objectives — as important as, or even more so than, learning labels or concepts. These attitudinal/temperamental factors significantly reduce and obstruct his ability to profit from his experiences and his ability to show his best capacities. Thus, Ronald can be reinforced not only for content that he learns, but for working longer and harder, and for trying alternatives when his first attempts fail.

8. Ronald's thinking ability may also be helped by relating his relatively weaker language skills to his visual–perceptual strength. Once he has mastered a visual–perceptual task, he can then be asked to talk more analytically about what he is doing. For example, once he shows that he can select a figure that matches a model from among many alternatives, attention can then be turned to helping him talk about what he did: "Why is that a good one? What is wrong with this other one?" As described above, it will first be necessary to model for him how to respond to these questions, and to induce imitation.

9. Ronald's already good ability to detect and complete sequences can be enhanced and elaborated into higher-level thinking skills by introducing and emphasizing planning experiences and verbal story sequences involving social interactions. Cooking is a good vehicle for talking about planning ("What do we need? what should we do first? Next? Last? What would happen if I did it this way instead of that way? Why do we need a plan?"). Following pictured story sequences with acting-out sequences may help to enhance Ronald's social interaction skills. It is especially important to try to link these "academic" exercises to Ronald's real-life interactions. His interactions can be observed, and he can be reminded: "Remember when we talked about that? What can you say when she says _____ ? What can you do now?" Similarly, his real-life interactions can be made into "academic" exercises (e.g., playing: "How can we get someone to play with us? What do we do after we get started?").

10. Interventions that have already been found to be successful with Ronald include provision of success; use of vocal intonations and shows of excitement to enhance meaning; provision of rhythms to enhance memory; copious provision of praise and encouragement; and contingency management ("Do this; then you can do _____ "). It is recommended that increased emphasis be placed on providing verbal elaborations and "bridges." Increased elaborations involve providing information regarding the materials and experiences with which he is engaged. For example, if he is working with Play-Doh, there can be talk about how soft it is, and that it has to be soft in order to be able to make so many things. "Bridging" involves connecting what Ronald is

doing at the time with either something he has done before or something he is anticipating in the future. The idea is to help him connect the perceptual (what he can see) with the conceptual (what he has to think about or imagine). For example: "Do you remember when we played this game before? When was another time when we had to make a plan like this?" At a more developed stage, he can be helped to engage in some more speculative ("what if") and cause-and-effect thinking. As always, when these more challenging demands are made, it is best to provide many models and to encourage imitation.

Case 2

Name: Jennifer Smith

Chronological Age: 7 years, 8 months

Reason for Referral: Jennifer's parents have specifically requested a dynamic assessment, rather than the more traditional type that Jennifer has had in the past. They are seeking qualitative rather than quantitative or placement information, to derive ideas regarding how she learns and how to teach her. The dynamic assessment model, in this case primarily based on the work of Feuerstein, involves intervening with the child during the course of the "testing" procedure (administered in test–intervene–retest format) to derive impressions regarding cognitive modifiability as well as hypotheses for intervention.

Background Information: Jennifer has been diagnosed as having cerebral palsy and developmental aphasia. Standardized testing results in scores within a high-trainable to low-educable retarded range, with somewhat higher levels in receptive language. She is currently enrolled in a program for trainable retarded children.

Procedures: The full Preschool Learning Assessment Device (PLAD) for use with young children was administered. Portions of other tests, both formal and informal, were administered utilizing just an "intervene" format. These included a variety of receptive and expressive vocabulary subtests, as well as an attempt at a matrices test.

Assessment Results: Jennifer is a warm, affectionate girl, who is interested in relating to and pleasing adults with whom she works. Because of her extreme difficulty with attention maintenance/distractibility, "work" accomplishment proceeded very slowly and sporadically, with frequent interruptions. It seems very difficult for Jennifer to sustain a thought and to inhibit her reactivity to what she sees and hears. Her behavior is also characterized by behavioral and verbal echolalia, as well as frequent perseveration. That is, she will often say and do what she hears and sees in direct imitation, and she will at times have difficulty inhibiting a behavior once begun. The echolalia appears to serve a combination of signaling difficulty with comprehension and providing additional time for her processing. The perseveration can be inhibited by telling her to stop (in fact, physically helping her to stop) and by redirecting her attention, preferably with a question such as "Can you make yourself stop? Now, what do we need to do?"

Jennifer also showed difficulty processing motor movements, particularly those involving motor planning. Similar to her delay between hearing and speaking was a delay between hearing and doing. At times she seemed at a loss to know how to start or how to sequence her movements. In these cases, it was necessary to provide maximum cueing, moving her through and verbalizing what needed to done.

Evidence of Jennifer's modifiability was often subtle, but nevertheless present. Although she did not make dramatic gains that were measurable in terms of scores on tests, she showed behavioral responsiveness that was very encouraging. These changes were accomplished by taking advantage of some naturally occurring "problem" situations, and by making problem solving her responsibility. For example, in one instance, Jennifer moved to a chair that was far removed from the assessor and the work. The assessor commented, "Is that a good place to sit? How can we do our work? What do you need to do?" and waited. After several seconds, Jennifer pulled the chair in which she was sitting to a position close to the assessor. In this way she and the assessor were satisfied: She got to keep her new seat, and the assessor got her closer to the work—a rather creative solution!

There were also definite improvements in her performance on the variety of tasks of the PLAD. This procedure involves administering the Triangles subtest of the Kaufman Assessment Battery for Children (K-ABC) as a pretest and posttest for the whole procedure. The "intervene" portion involves three activities incorporating cognitive prerequisites related to the Triangles subtest, each with its own pretest and posttest. During the first activity, a request to draw a child, Jennifer produced a series of separated circles. She was able to progress to inclusion of lines with her circles, although these still remained disconnected. The intervention that promoted the greatest integration was to allow her to imitate a simply drawn figure that was previously reviewed in detail. It was necessary to take time to practice making the shapes involved in the figure. When allowed to imitate, she was able to approximate a more recognizable result.

The second task involved building steps with 10 cubes. Jennifer was able to recognize and label the model built for her, and was able to produce meaningful conversation about steps. Block building is particularly difficult for her because of her mild palsy, but she is clearly able to build towers and related constructions, with some messiness and slippage. Integration of the discrete parts was a significant obstruction for her in this task, and she did best when the structural outline was provided for her and when she filled this in with her blocks. There is a pattern of difficulty dealing with a "blank space" that relates not only to Jennifer's problems with integration, but to her difficulty with motor planning as well (i.e., not knowing just where or how to begin). Allowing her to imitate a model can be helpful, but Jennifer needs specific attention to learn how to profit from looking at a model. She needs encouragement to use her eyes to guide her movements and to find out what to do, and to help her know what to look for when she looks. This is often best followed by moving her through the task (literally moving her hands), while verbalizing what she can do in a way that she can remember (short, simple, repeated statements).

On the third task, parquetry, Jennifer showed the most improvement. On the pretest, she had no idea how to proceed, and made no attempt to reproduce the model (a design of a rocket). On the posttest, she clearly placed the middle red block appropriately to match the model, and checked back to the model while doing so. Although the whole figure did not recreate the model picture, her production was much more organized and integrated. The pieces all touched, and were organized by color, approximating the verticality of the rocket she was trying to create. What seemed to help her in this task was giving her experience with placing the blocks directly on top of the picture, while talking her through the task solution and providing physical structure for her placement of her pieces. She also profited from induction of meaning about the model — that is, eliciting from her what the picture looked like, followed by elaboration about rockets. This is the task for which she produced remote recall, coming in the next day with recollection of the rocket she had worked on the previous day.

On the final posttest of the K-ABC Triangles, Jennifer showed improved focus and an increase in the deliberateness and goal-directedness of her actions. She seemed more assured about what to do, and was able to turn the small triangles in a variety of directions to achieve a solution. Although she proceeded in trial-and-error fashion, she showed flexibility in her ability to change the relationship of the pieces in search of a solution. Jennifer had difficulty responding to two simultaneous concepts (color plus shape), but she did successfully produce two shapes during the posttest phase.

Jennifer showed difficulty with color concepts throughout the assessment. Her father reported successful color matching at home, and she spontaneously correctly labeled red when not directly asked, but secure color matching or naming was never elicited. Jennifer often sought to sit on the assessor's lap, and this did seem to help her focus. She is able to recognize her correct solutions, and shows delight when she succeeds.

Jennifer has a very skittish response to difficulty; she offers a multitude of excuses, requests, and distractions. She is helped by being asked whether she needs help at these times ("Is this hard? Can I help you?"). The need to complete tasks and the setting of contingencies for accomplishing this is important for her. This needs to be stated explictly for and then elicited from her ("What do you need to do before you have a snack?").

Jennifer offered many instances of good verbal communication during the course of the assessment. She was able to express her needs and desires, and spoke in many single sentences of five to six words. Most impressive was her spontaneous comment at the end of the first day of work with her, when she said, "I need to think about that." Somehow, the point of the whole interaction seemed to register and be understood.

Jennifer's use of her eyes continues to raise questions about the adequacy of her vision. She held her eyes very close to the materials, and used her eyes relatively ineffectively. This may warrant a recheck. If her vision is not adequate, this may be one reason for her high level of distractibility.

Jennifer moves her body a great deal, and has a hard time remaining still. During the assessment, she responded briefly but appropriately to inducements to "fix your body so you can do your work," or more simply to "Are you ready? Get your body ready." This placed the problem solving in her hands. That is, she was not directly told how to sit or what to do. She had to do her own problem solving to respond, and she did this quite well. Occupational therapy may be helpful in addressing Jennifer's frequent position changes, as well as her motor planning difficulty. Jennifer is at a good age to profit from sensory-motor integration therapy.

Recommendations:

1. Two handouts are attached to this report that elaborate on Feuerstein's core concept of "mediated learning experience" (MLE).* The components of MLE are thought by many to represent the crux of good teaching practices. Especially important to helping children become good thinkers and problem solvers are the components of "transcendence" and "planning," although all of the components should be present somewhere during the course of an extended teaching interaction. Transcendence involves "bridging" what is currently seen

---

*Note to the reader: These handouts are not provided here.

or experienced by the child with experiences the child has had before or may anticipate in the future — that is, helping the child to make connections between what is seen and what must be imagined. This can be done with questions such as "When did we do this before?" or "What was another time when we had to make a plan?" Planning involves helping the child to think of the best sequence and strategies for the task (e.g., "First look at color, then shape"). These may have to be asked rhetorically (i.e., asked and then answered by the adult). However, the questions need to be asked even if the child is at first unable to respond, in order to create a disequilibrium and readiness that help to engage the child's attention and to promote the child's ability to develop the need to think.

2. Jennifer's vision should be rechecked, and an optometrist should perhaps be consulted regarding the value of "vision training." This should only be done in relation to a specific eye problem (e.g., weak muscles), and not with the idea that this training will teach her how to read.

3. An occupational therapy assessment should be performed; therapy, if deemed helpful, should be provided by an experienced pediatric occupational therapist who is certified in sensory–motor integration therapy. Related to this, and in consultation with an occupational or physical therapist, Jennifer might perhaps be involved in therapeutic horseback riding. There is some promising evidence that horseback riding can be helpful to children with cerebral palsy. Jennifer will need help to deal with her fearfulness. Swimming may be another activity that will facilitate her sensory–motor functioning.

4. If vision is securely ruled out as a major source of distraction, a trial of stimulant medication may be helpful to try to increase Jennifer's ability to maintain attention. If this option is considered, it should be done in consultation with a physician who is experienced in this area, and who will provide adequate follow-up.

5. Many areas are in the process of adopting Feuerstein's approaches to assessment and education. A call to the state department of education may be helpful in locating individuals in the school system or the who are knowledgeable about this approach, and who may serve as teacher consultants for Jennifer.

6. Some educational strategies that have been built into mediationally based curricula and that have been found to be helpful in promoting cognitive development include the following:

a. Beginning the day with "planning time." This involves discussing the sequence of activities for the day; these are checked off as they occur. For each activity, the teacher should discuss with the children the materials that are needed and the best sequence and strategies to follow. After each activity, they should discuss what was done (and, if there were any glitches, what went wrong).

b. Ending the day with "summary time" to review the day's activities. As in any activity, the teacher should try to elicit as much as possible from the children.

c. Organizing the curriculum to include not only content, but processes as well (e.g., making a plan; comparing; self-regulation). All the activities of the day can address the processes of the day. The processes should be explicitly stated and reviewed throughout the day, so that the children will be able to state what they have learned by the end of the day in terms of both process and content.

d. Building "bridges" into all activities, relating the content in school to experiences of the children in other contexts. These need to be preplanned so that the teacher can fill in gaps when the children draw a blank (e.g., "Did we do anything like this before? Do you do anything like this at home? When is another time that we need to _____ ?").

Case 3

Name: Bob Johnson

Chronological Age: 6 years, 7 months

Reason for Referral: Bob will be entering a regular kindergarten program in the fall. Bob's parents have specifically requested a dynamic assessment to learn about his "learning style," strengths and weaknesses, and directions for future educational programming. Traditional assessments have been carried out in the past and are available from his parents.

Background Information: Bob lives with his parents and his $1\frac{1}{2}$ year old sister. He has participated in a preschool since the age of $3\frac{1}{2}$ years. Early history is significant for diagnosis of Down's syndrome, open heart surgery (age $1\frac{1}{2}$), and eye surgery (age $4\frac{1}{2}$). His heart surgery was considered successful, and he has no sequelae. The eye surgery was to keep his eye from turning outward, which resulted in Bob's tilting his head to improve his acuity; his vision is currently reported as adequate, with occasional turning in of his eye. Bob may have a mild hearing deficiency, and this is being monitored by his speech therapist; his hearing appears adequate for conversation and classroom teaching. Bob adjusted well to his preschool, and was noted for good social interaction with peers. His father, who brought him for the assessment, observes generally low energy level.

While in preschool, Bob received services from speech, occupational, and physical therapists. He also received special education services from a teacher who has some familiarity with the Cognitive Education Curriculum for Young Children, developed at the Kennedy Center of Vanderbilt University. She will continue to work with him in the afternoons, following Bob's attendance at a regular kindergarten program in the mornings. She will also serve as a liaison with the teachers and therapists, with particular attention to ensuring consistency among the cognitive components of his experiences.

Procedures:

- Parent interview
- File review
- Goodman Lock Box (a play assessment procedure)
- Preschool Learning Assessment Device
- Children's Analogical Test of Modifiability
- Frame Test of Cognitive Modifiability

The last three procedures are "dynamic"; that is, they are administered in a test–intervene–retest format, with focus on the intervention aspects that reveal strengths and weaknesses of cognitive processing, responsiveness to mediation, and an array of trial interventions.

Assessment Results: Bob is a small, blond-haired boy, who relates in a very warm, friendly way. He communicates freely in a telegraphic manner, with some need for help to translate his articulation. His ability to express his thoughts is not up to the level of his ability to understand or conceptualize his ideas, and at times he shows awareness of and frustration with this. He continues to enhance his communication with gestures (sometimes signs). Bob demonstrates good memory of what is said to him and is able to relate salient ideas and sequences of his experiences. He shows awareness of the concepts of past and future time and of numbers, although he is not always precise in his labeling of these concepts. He is enthusiastic and fun to work with.

During the assessment, Bob would typically begin new work eagerly and receptively. However, when confronted with difficulty, he would decide that he was "tired" and "done," and then could at times be difficult to re-engage. However, he was more often a good worker, and it was possible to carry out a wide variety of tasks with him. He could be worked with for periods of at least 1 to $1\frac{1}{2}$ hours. He demonstrated a very good conceptual knowledge base. He not only could name many things that he saw, but could name many from his internalized repertory as well. He was also able to anticipate consequences of some behaviors (e.g., that a large pile of blocks might fall or that a bouncing ball might break objects).

Bob's interaction with the Goodman Lock Box, a play assessment procedure, demonstrated his high level of organization and ability to engage in symbolic play. He managed to open all but the two most difficult locks; therefore, even in view of his fine motor delays, he was able to obtain a level of performance above an "at-risk" status on the motor component of this task. The procedure could not be scored formally, because Bob was apparently waiting for permission to remove the toys, and in so doing considerably delayed his play interactions while engaging in repetitive unlocking and relocking behavior. However, once it was realized that he awaited "permission," he readily interacted with the materials, showed ability to initiate and maintain a stable organizational pattern, knew how to play with each of the toys, and demonstrated many appropriate toy combinations. Of special note was that the symbolic level of Bob's play was greatest with the Play-Doh — that is, when the play material was lowest in definition. With toys that had a more clearly defined use, he carried out that function quickly, but was not stimulated to apply his imagination. With the Play-Doh, he developed a prolonged story sequence involving a castle, a bridge, and a meal, molding pieces to represent each of the ideas he expressed. Bob was also able to maintain independent play throughout most of the feedback time of about 1 hour.

On the dynamic assessment tasks, Bob demonstrated several things. First was his high degree of responsiveness to intervention. In virtually every instance, Bob was able to make positive gains, and always in the direction promoted by the intervention. It was never necessary to work on his knowledge base; he always had the basic concepts necessary for the tasks. He would become overwhelmed by too many elements, and paring down the number of items or objects to deal with was a successful strategy for him. In this case, his perception of "too many" obstructed his attention and his ability to analyze the details of what he perceived. For example, what at first appeared to be difficulty with demonstrating spatial orientation turned out to be difficulty with processing too many pieces. When the number of items was reduced, he was successful in showing good spatial awareness.

Bob also readily showed the ability to use concepts and strategies offered to him and to internalize these as self-talk, used to guide his own behavior. Concepts that personalized abstract relationships were particularly useful, such as calling a category a "family." Using the classificatory family concept, Bob showed himself able to utilize two simultaneous concepts (namely, color and size). He also quickly responded to reminders to "look at the model," and was able to improve his performance when he did this, suggesting that he knew what to notice when he looked.

Bob's motor delay showed potential for improvement via a cognitive route. His drawings tended to be perseverative, impulsive, and imprecise, with the motor product not adequately representing his cognitive concept. However, with discussion and demonstration of the need to form and carry out a plan, in addition to specific practice of fast and slow movements (with the motor behavior following the cognitive decision — i.e., decide to move fast, then move fast; decide to move slowly, then move slowly), he was able to make dramatic changes in figure drawing over a 3-day period of time. His first drawing of a "fireman" was a straight line with a repetitive series of criss-crossed horizontal lines, resulting in no resemblance to a human figure. His second drawing, although still not figure-like or well differentiated, did incorporate multiple circles and dots, both of which were part of the intervention discussion (he had decided dots were to be used for fingers). The third drawing, while inverted, was recognizably figure-like, with a clearly drawn circle for a head, two legs and two arms in appropriate positions, and multiple fingers (now lines) crisscrossing the arms. Finally, almost as an afterthought, Bob drew a circle head on top of an oblong body in the correct orientation, seeming to surprise himself with his success. His need was to slow down his motoric impulsivity with increased cognitive control over his movements.

It was also possible to help Bob deal with his feelings of being overwhelmed by too many pieces through improving his ability to engage in part–whole analysis. His difficulty seemed to be "not seeing the trees for the forest," rather than vice versa. He would see a lot of things and seem to say to himself (or others), "This is too hard," and be unable to look for subparts that he could tackle. This was particularly apparent when he was working with parquetry designs. Helping him to make a plan and decide where to start, and then holding him to that sequence, moving him systematically from segment to segment, seemed to break his "too hard" gestalt; when re-presented with the original design, he could quickly zero in on a subpart and proceed with that, rather than reject the whole.

Bob was found to need some work in the area of increasing the flexibility of his response to change. When a minor change was made, such as rotating a parquetry design he had mastered, he responded as if a major change had ensued. This suggested difficulty with perceiving and analyzing the elements in terms of "what changed" and "what remained the same." It is possible that in other areas as well, what may seem like a minor change to others may be experienced by Bob as much more major. If this is the case, he may need not only preparatory warnings of imminent changes, but specific help with perceiving and recognizing similarities and differences, and help with using the similarities as clues to help him know what to do.

Summary and Recommendations: Bob has been provided with rich and extensive experiences, and has made good progress in response to these. He is quite modifiable and clearly a learner. He needs to be provided with sufficient time and practice to realize and solidify his gains. New learning is best introduced early and briefly during his most alert and receptive moments, allowing him time to move in and out of his willingness to risk exposure to the unknown. At times it is necessary to follow his lead and to try to fit the learning objectives into the object of his attention, rather than to insist on his total compliance; this requires flexibility and inventiveness on the part of the adults working with him. Effort needs to be spent in trying to prevent his experiencing frustration (e.g., by simplifying materials, reducing number of items, etc.), to avoid the need to try to re-engage him after he has experienced frustration.

Attention to the need for flexibility and ability to deal with changes from expected routines and patterns can be addressed as specific learning objectives for Bob. Once he learns how to do something, he can be encouraged to "do it another way," or "Let's change it and see what happens" can be suggested. Subskills he will need in order to handle this include application of "same" and "different" concepts to increasingly complex experiences. He can then be asked "What is the same?" and "What is different?" about the changed picture, object, game, or experience. He can also be encouraged to make the changes, and then to discuss what he has changed and what he has left the same. (As in any new learning, the adult will need to do more modeling, explaining, and demonstrating at the beginning.)

During the assessment, Bob responded very well to practicing "slow" and "fast" self-control, applied to drawing, ball throwing, and walking. The idea that "fast" sometimes leads to mistakes was emphasized, and it was pointed out to him that he draws better when he slows down. Adults working with Bob should be aware that it is best for him first to say what he will do, and then to do it. When drawing, he can draw fast and slow lines or shapes, and then be asked to do a more complex drawing with the reminder: "How do you need to do this? Fast or slow?" He can play a ball-rolling game by saying "I roll the ball fast/slow" and then do it. This can be elaborated by having him roll the ball to hit a picture or object of a new concept to be learned (e.g., "I roll the ball fast to the triangle"). His increased self-regulation may also help to improve development of one-to-one correspondence in counting; it may also help to have him move the object he is counting as he counts it.

Bob's symbolic play appears facilitated by materials that are not well defined in and of themselves. Continued encouragement of his use of materials such as Play-Doh is recommended.

It is helpful to be alert for naturally occurring "problems" and to pose questions to stimulate Bob's thinking about the problem: "See what happened here? What can we do?" Then evaluation of possible solutions can be considered. Many ordinary incidents can be reinterpreted as problems to be solved (e.g., "Uh-oh, I only have one serving of cereal left, and two of you want cereal; what can we do?"). Many times, a problem can be posed rhetorically; the important thing is to ask questions to promote Bob's active thinking and to provide a model for problem solving, which can also be done as adult self-talk in front of him.

Bob's ploy of being "tired" can be reinterpreted to him as follows: "I think you are really saying that this looks hard. Can you help me find a way to make it easy? Let's try it this way and see if that helps."

Some additional activities that have been developed for a summer program, using the Kennedy Center's Cognitive Education Curriculum for Young Children, will be forwarded.

APPENDIX III.A. Dynamic Assessment Recording Form

Name: _____   Date: _____   Location:_____

Examiner: _____   Task: (see Appendix III.B) _____

Learner characteristics/ processes (check if required by task)	Pretest	Intervention	Posttest	Presence	Change

Knowledge base
- Vocabulary
- Information
- Skills

Arousal/attention
- Arousal rate (hyper-/hypo-/ optimal)
- Attention
  Orienting
  Selective
  Divided
  Sustained
  Capacity
  Modality effect?

Coding/analysis (simultaneous vs. successive)
- Perception
  Stimulus detection
  Feature discrimination
  Stimulus recognition
  Stimulus comparisons
  Perceptual strategy
- Memory
  Storage
    Short-term
    Long-term
  Retrieval

Planning
- Problem recognition
- Problem definition
- Strategy determination/
  selection
- Enactment/application
- Self-regulation/
  impulse control
- Evaluation/analysis
- Adjustment/modification

Output
- Modality effects
  (e.g., verbal, motor)
- Content effects
- Qualitative effects
  (e.g., organization,
  structure, precision)

APPENDIX III.B. Analysis of the Task

1. Name of the task:
2. Content of the task (specify knowledge base required and materials involved):

3. Processes required:

4. Operations involved (e.g., identification, comparison, analogical reasoning, deductive reasoning, inductive reasoning, categorization, seriation, multiplication, other):

5. Modality (or modalities) involved (e.g., auditory, visual, tactile, kinesthetic, verbal, pictorial, numerical, figural, symbolic, graphic, other):

6. Complexity:
   Units of information: High   10 9 8 7 6 5 4 3 2 1   Low
   Degree of familiarity: High   5 4 3 2 1   Low
   Comment:

7. Abstraction:
   Abstract   5 4 3 2 1   Concrete
   Comment:

8. Efficiency:
   Speed: Fast   5 4 3 2 1   Slow
   Precision: High   5 4 3 2 1   Low
   Comment:

9. Additional comments:

APPENDIX III.C. Summary of Dynamic Assessment Results

Child's Name: _____ Date: _____ Assessor:_____

Task: _____ Situation:_____

1. What relevant processes are intact?

2. What relevant processes are weak but evident?

3. What relevant processes need attention?

4. How responsive was the child to intervention?

Very	Moderately	Slightly	Not at all
•	•	•	•

Comment:

5. How intense an effort was required to induce change?

Minimal	Low moderate	High moderate	Extreme
•	•	•	•

Comment:

6. What interventions:
   a. appeared to work?

   b. were tried and did not work?

   c. were not tried, but might work?

7. Was there any indication of transfer of learning?

   Yes __   Some __   No __

   Describe:

8. Overall impressions and additional comments:

APPENDIX III.D. Individualized Educational Program

Child's Name: _____ Date: _____ Area: Cognition

_____ is now able to:

_____ needs to learn to:

Recommended interventions for each objective:

How each objective will be evaluated and by whom:

When work will begin:
(Indicate next to each objective the date when each has been accomplished)

APPENDIX III.E. PLAD Procedural Checklist

Child's Name: _____ Date of PLAD:_____

Examiner:_____

__ Administer K-ABC pretest (Triangles subtest).
__ Introduce PLAD procedure to child.
__ Discuss initial observations re functions to be worked on.
__ Administer figure drawing pretest, presenting materials in problem-solving way.
__ Include human figure puzzle in mediation.
__ Include child instructing examiner in mediation.
__ Include individualized needs in mediation.
__ Administer figure drawing posttest.
__ Compare pretest and posttest with child.
__ Rediscuss progress and needs vis-à-vis cognitive functions.
__ Administer block steps pretest, presenting materials in problem-solving way.
__ Discuss cognitive functions to be addressed.
__ Mediate block steps task.
__ Administer block steps posttest.
__ Compare pretest and posttest of block steps task.
__ Administer parquetry pretest, presenting materials in problem-solving way.
__ Discuss cognitive functions to be addressed.
__ Include choice between two designs in mediation.
__ Include movement from blocks on design, to blocks off design onto outlined figure, to blocks onto blank page in mediation.
__ Include mediation of individualized needs.
__ Administer parquetry posttest.
__ Compare pretest and posttest with child.
__ Review cognitive functions addressed and progress on these.
__ Note indications of spontaneous applications of what was learned, as well as any original contributions of child.
__ Note behaviors of examiner that facilitated or obstructed child's learning.
__ Administer K-ABC posttest (Triangles subtest)

APPENDIX III.F. Lesson Planning Sheet

Child's Name: _____ Teacher's Name: _____ Date:_____

1. What is the task?

2. What instructions will you give?

3. What does the child actually have to do?

4. How will you present the materials and break down the task?

5. How will you facilitate the child's attention?

6. How will you promote memory?

7. How will you promote transfer?

8. When can you work on this with the child?

9. How can you build this into other (including group) lessons?

APPENDIX III.G. Record of Teaching Sessions

Child's Name: _____ Date: _____ Teacher:_____

Task: _____ Situation:_____

1. Objective worked on:

2. Interventions tried:

3. Child's response:

4. Next time:

5. Comments:

APPENDIX III.H. Curriculum-Based Dynamic Assessment Competency Checklist

Each of the following is evaluated on this scale:

Complete mastery	High mastery	Median mastery	Minimal mastery	No mastery
•	•	•	•	•
4	3	2	1	0

1. Task selected is (a) appropriate for child's level and (b) an important component of the curriculum:
   Rating:
   a.
   b.
   Comment:

2. Task is appropriately divided into three equal and testable parts:
   Rating:
   Comment:

3. Processes indicated are appropriate to the task:
   Rating:
   Comment:

4. Teacher (a) plans lessons ahead and (b) anticipates how to intervene in areas outlined on the lesson plan sheets:
   Rating:
   a.
   b.
   Comment:

5. Teacher administers pre- and posttests appropriately and without intervention:
   Rating:
   Comment:

6. Teacher interacts in terms of the MLE components as outlined on the MLE Rating Scale:
   Rate teacher on Rating Scale:
   Comment:

7. Teacher records appropriate notes during the course of the assessment:
   Rating:
   Comment:

8. Teacher (a) completes summary form immediately after the assessment and (b) with appropriate information:
   Rating:
      a.
      b.
   Comment:

9. Teacher develops relevant objectives based on the information from the assessment:
   Rating:
   Comment:

                     Rater's Name:
                     Date of Rating:

Resources

Information about the Learning Potential Assessment Device (LPAD) and future LPAD workshops is available from Professor Reuven Feuerstein at this address:

Hadassah-WIZO-Canada Research Institute
6 Karmon Street, P.O. Box 3160
Beit Hakerem
Jerusalem 96308
Israel

As of this writing, a course on dynamic assessment procedures, including the LPAD, will be taught by Dr. Kevin Keane at Columbia University's Teachers College in New York City. There are others around the country who are experienced LPAD assessors and instructors, such as Dr. H. Carl Haywood at Vanderbilt University, and Dr. Asa Hilliard at Georgia State University.

Dr. Milton Budoff's specific instruments, as well as results of numerous research studies, are available from Dr. Budoff at this address:

Research Institute for Educational Problems, Inc.
29 Ware Street
Cambridge, MA 02138

Information and materials related to preschool procedures developed by Dr. David Tzuriel and Dr. Pnina S. Klein can be obtained from Dr. Tzuriel at this address:

School of Education
Bar Ilan University
Ramat Gan 52100
Israel

Information regarding the preschool procedures developed by Dr. M. Susan Burns can be obtained from Dr. Burns at this address:

> Department of Education
> Tulane University
> Alcee Fortier Building
> New Orleans, LA 70118

Information regarding the *European Journal of Psychology of Education* can be obtained from this address:

> Instituto Superior de Psicologia Aplicada
> Rua Jardin do Tabaco, 44
> 1100 Lisboa
> Portugal

Information regarding dynamic assessment instruments available in Germany can be obtained from one of these addresses:

> The Psychodiagnostic Center
> Department of Psychology
> Humboldt University
> Oranienburgerstrasse 18
> Berlin 1080
> Germany

> or

> Test Center
> Dr. Hogrefe Publishing House
> (Gottingen), D-7000
> Darmlerstrasse 40
> Stuttgart 50
> Germany

Information regarding learning tests designed and/or published in The Netherlands can be obtained from Professor J. H. M. Hamers at this address:

> Department of Special Education
> University of Utrecht
> Heidelberglaan 1
> P.O. Box 80.140
> 3508 TC Utrecht
> The Netherlands

The Test of Children's Learning Ability, published in Great Britain, can be obtained from one of these addresses:

National Foundation for Educational Research (NFER) Publishing
    Company, Ltd.
Darville House
2 Oxford Road East
Windsor, Berkshire SL4 1DF
England

or

Humanities Press, Inc.
Atlantic Highlands, NJ 07716

There are a number of researchers in Canada actively involved in development and investigation of dynamic assessment procedures. Two primary sources for information on Canadian involvement in this area are the following:

Dr. Peter J. Gamlin
The Ontario Institute for Studies in Education
252 Bloor Street W.
Toronto, Ontario M5S 1V6
Canada

and

Dr. Marilyn Samuels
The Learning Centre
2315 First Avenue, N.W.
Calgary, Alberta T2N 2N9
Canada

Information regarding the Cognitive Education Curriculum for Young Children can be obtained from Dr. H. Carl Haywood at this address:

Vanderbilt University
Kennedy Center
Box 9, Peabody Station
Nashville, TN 37203

Parquetry materials for the PLAD can be purchased from the following:

Developmental Learning Materials (DLM)
P.O. Box 4000
One DLM Park
Allen, TX 75002
(800-527-4747)

Finally, there are now two journals dedicated to the publication of information related to dynamic assessment and cognitive education. The first of these is the *International Journal of Dynamic Assessment and Instruction*. Subscription information about this journal is available from this address:

Captus Press, Inc.
York University Campus
4700 Keele Street
North York, Ontario M3J 1P3
Canada

The other journal is the *International Journal of Cognitive Education and Mediated Learning*. Subscription information is available from one of these addresses:

Dr. Martha Coulter
University of South Florida
College of Public Health
13301 Bruce B. Downs Boulevard
Tampa, FL 33613-3899

or

International Journal of Cognitive Education and Mediated Learning
6/7 Hockley Hill
Birmingham B18 5AA
England

References

Anastasi, A. (1981). Diverse effects of training on tests of academic intelligence. In B. F. Green (Ed.), *New directions for testing and measurement: No. 11. Issues in testing — coaching, disclosure, and ethnic bias.* San Francisco: Jossey-Bass.

Arthur, G. (1945). *Stencil Design Test 1 of the Arthur Point Scale of Performance Tests.* New York: Psychological Corporation.

Babad, E., & Bashi, J. (1975). *Final report: An educational test of the validity of learning potential measurement* (RIEPrint No. 91). Cambridge, MA: Research Institute for Educational Problems.

Babad, E. Y., & Budoff, M. (1974). Sensitivity and validity of learning potential measurement in three levels of ability. *Journal of Educational Psychology, 66,* 439–447.

Bailey, D. B., Jr. (1981). Investigation of learning measures as screening procedures with kindergartners. *Psychology in the Schools, 18,* 489–495.

Bakeman, R., & Brown, J. V. (1980). Early interaction: Consequences for social and mental development at three years. *Child Development, 51,* 437–447.

Baldwin, R. L., Cole, R. E., & Baldwin, C. P. (Eds.). (1982). Parental pathology, family interaction, and the competence of the child in school. *Monographs of the Society for Research in Child Development, 47*(5, Serial No. 197).

Ballester, L. E. (1984). *Feuerstein's model of cognitive functioning applied to preschool children: A study of the relationship between specific cognitive strategies and learning.* Unpublished doctoral dissertation, Temple University.

Bayley, N., & Schaefer, E. S. (1964). Correlations of maternal and child behaviors with the development of mental abilities: Data from the Berkeley Growth Study. *Monographs of the Society for Research in Child Development, 29*(16, Serial No. 97).

Bell, R. Q. (1979). Parent, child, and reciprocal influences. *American Psychologist, 34,* 821–826.

Bethge, H., Carlson, J. S., & Wiedl, K. H. (1982). The effects of dynamic assessment procedures on Raven Matrices performance, visual search behavior, test anxiety, and test orientation. *Intelligence, 6,* 89–97.

Binet, A., & Simon, T. (1980). *The development of intelligence in children.* Nashville, TN: Williams. (Original work published 1916)

Bornstein, M. H., & Tamis-LeMonda, C. S. (1989). Maternal responsiveness and cognitive development. In M. H. Bornstein (Ed.), *New directions for child development: No. 43. Maternal responsiveness: Characteristics and consequences.* San Francisco: Jossey-Bass.

Bortner, M., & Birch, H. G. (1969). Cognitive capacity and cognitive competence. *American Journal of Mental Deficiency, 74,* 735–744.

Bradley, R. H. (1989). HOME measurement of maternal responsiveness. In M. H. Bornstein (Ed.), New *directions for child development: No. 43. Maternal responsiveness: Characteristics and consequences.* San Francisco: Jossey-Bass.

Bradley, R. H., & Caldwell, B. M. (1976). The relation of infants' home environments to mental test performance at fifty-four months: A follow-up study. *Child Development, 47,* 1172–1174.

Bradley, R. H., Caldwell, B. M., & Rock, S. L. (1988). Home environment and school performance: A ten-year follow-up and examination of three models of environmental action. *Child Development, 59,* 852–867.

Bransford, J. D., Delclos, V. R., Vye, N. J., Burns, M. S., & Hasselbring, T. S. (1986). *Improving the quality of assessment and instruction: Roles for dynamic assessment.* Nashville, TN: John F. Kennedy Center for Research on Education and Human Development, Vanderbilt University.

Bryant, N. R. (1982). *Preschool children's learning and transfer of matrices problems: A study of proximal development.* Unpublished master's thesis, University of Illinois.

Budoff, M. (1987a). The validity of learning potential assessment. In C. S. Lidz (Ed.), *Dynamic assessment: An interactional approach to evaluating learning potential.* New York: Guilford Press.

Budoff, M. (1987b). Measures for assessing learning potential. In C. S. Lidz (Ed.), *Dynamic assessment: An interactional approach to evaluating learning potential.* New York: Guilford Press.

Budoff, M., & Allen, P. (1978). *The utility of a learning potential test with substantially mentally retarded students: Application of a formboard version of the Raven Progressive Matrices (Sets A, AB, B)* (RIEPrint No. 110). Cambridge, MA: Research Institute for Educational Problems.

Budoff, M., & Corman, L. (1973). *The effectiveness of a group training procedure on the Raven learning potential measure with children of diverse racial and socio-economic backgrounds* (RIEPrint No. 58). Cambridge, MA: Research Institute for Educational Problems.

Budoff, M., Corman, L., & Gimon, A. (1976). An educational test of learning potential assessment with Spanish-speaking youth. *Interamerican Journal of Psychology, 10,* 13–24.

Budoff, M., & Hamilton, J. (1976). Optimizing test performance of the moderately and severely mentally retarded. *American Journal of Mental Deficiency, 81,* 49–57.

Budoff, M., Meskin, J., & Harrison, R. G. (1971). An educational test of the learning potential hypothesis. *American Journal of Mental Deficiency, 76,* 159–169.

Burns, M. S. (1980). *Preschool children's approach and performance on cognitive tasks.* Unpublished master's thesis, Vanderbilt University.

Burns, M. S. (1985). *Comparison of "graduated prompt" and "mediational" dynamic assessment and static assessment with young children.* Unpublished doctoral dissertation, Vanderbilt University.

Burns, M. S., Haywood, H. C., Delclos, V. R., & Siewert, L. (1985). *Young children's problem-solving strategies: An observational study* (Alternative Assessments of Handicapped Children, Technical Report No. 1). Nashville, TN: John F. Kennedy Center for Research on Education and Human Development, Vanderbilt University.

Burns, M. S., Vye, N. J., Bransford, J. D., Delclos, V., & Ogan, T. (1987). Static and dynamic measures of learning in young handicapped children. *Diagnostique, 12,* 59–73.

Camp, B. W. (1973). Psychometric tests and learning in severely disabled readers. *Journal of Learning Disabilities, 6,* 512–517.

Camp, B. W., Swift, W. J., & Swift, E. W. (1982). Authoritarian parental attitudes and cognitive functioning in preschool children. *Psychological Reports, 50,* 1023–1026.

Campione, J. C., & Brown, A. L. (1990). Guided learning and transfer: Implications for approaches to assessment. In N. Frederiksen, R. Glaser, A. Lesgold, & M. G. Shafto (Eds.), *Diagnostic monitoring of skill and knowledge acquisition.* Hillsdale, NJ: Erlbaum.

Campione, J. C., Brown, A. L., & Bryant, N. R. (1985). Individual differences in learning and memory. In R. J. Sternberg (Ed.), *Human abilities: An information processing approach.* New York: W. H. Freeman.

Campione, J. C., Brown, A. L., Ferrara, R. A., Jones, R. S., & Steinberg, E. (1985). Differences between retarded and non-retarded children in transfer following equivalent learning performances: Breakdowns in flexible use of information. *Intelligence, 9,* 297–315.

Carew, J. V. (1980). Experience and the development of intelligence in young children at home and in day care. *Monographs of the Society for Research in Child Development, 45* (6–7, Serial No. 187).

Carlson, J. S., & Wiedl, K. H. (1980). Applications of a dynamic testing approach in intelligence assessment: Empirical results and theoretical formulations. *Zeitschrift für Differentiele und Diagnostische Psychologie, 1,* 303–318.

Clarke-Stewart, K. A. (1973). Interactions between mothers and their young children: Characteristics and consequences. *Monographs of the Society for Research in Child Development, 38*(6–7, Serial No. 153).

Clarke-Stewart, K. A. (1988). Parents' effects on children's development: A decade of progress? *Journal of Applied Developmental Psychology, 9,* 41–84.

Collins, A. (1990). Reformulating testing to measure learning and thinking. In N. Frederiksen, R. Glaser, A. Lesgold, & M. G. Shafto (Eds.), *Diagnostic monitoring of skill and knowledge acquisition.* Hillsdale, NJ: Erlbaum.

Collins, M., Carnine, D., & Gersten, R. (1987). Elaborated corrective feedback and the acquisition of reasoning skills: A study of computer-assisted instruction. *Exceptional Children, 54,* 254–262.

Cormier, P., Carlson, J. S., & Das, J. P. (no date). *Planning ability and cognitive performance: The compensatory effects of dynamic assessment.* Unpublished manuscript, University of California–Riverside, School of Education.

Cox, A. D., Puckering, C., Pound, A., & Mills, M. (1987). The impact of maternal depression in young children. *Journal of Child Psychology and Psychiatry, 28,* 917–928.

Das, J. P. (1984). Simultaneous and successive processing in children with reading disability. *Topics in Language Disorders, 4,* 34–47.

Day, J. D., & Hall, L. K. (1987). Cognitive assessment, intelligence, and instruction. In J. D. Day & J. G. Borkowski (Eds.), *Intelligence and exceptionality: New directions for theory, assessment, and instructional practices.* Norwood, NJ: Ablex.

Dearborn, W. F. (1921). Intelligence and its measurement. *Journal of Educational Psychology, 12,* 210–212.

Delclos, V. R., Burns, M. S., & Kulewicz, S. J. (1987). Effects of dynamic assessment on teachers' expectations of handicapped children. *American Educational Research Journal, 24,* 325–336.

DeLoache, J. S., & DeMendoza, O. A. (1987). Joint picturebook interactions of mothers and 1-year-old children. *British Journal of Developmental Psychology, 5,* 111–123.

DeWeerdt, E. H. (1927). A study of the improvability of fifth grade school children in certain mental functions. *Journal of Educational Psychology, 18,* 547–557.

Embretson, S. E. (1987). Improving the measurement of spatial aptitude by dynamic testing. *Intelligence, 11,* 333–358.

Epstein, A. S. (1980). *Assessing the child development information needed by adolescent parents with very young children.* Washington, DC: Department of Health, Education and Welfare.

Estes, W. K. (1981). Intelligence and learning. In M. P. Friedman, J. P. Das, & N. O'Connor (Eds.), *Intelligence and learning.* New York: Plenum.

Estrada, P., Arsenio, W., Hess, R., & Holloway, S. (1987). Affective quality of the mother–child relationship: Longitudinal consequences for children's school-relevant cognitive functioning. *Developmental Psychology, 23,* 210–215.

Falik, L. H. (1989, August 6–8). *A mediational matrix: Observing and coding the mediational encounter.* Paper presented at the Second International Conference on Mediated Learning Experience, Knoxville, TN.

Farran, D. C., & Haskins, R. (1980). Reciprocal influence in the social interactions of mothers and three-year-old children from different socioeconomic backgrounds. *Child Development, 51,* 780–791.

Feshbach, N. D. (1973). Cross-cultural studies of teaching styles in four-year-olds and their mothers. In A. D. Pick (Ed.), *Minnesota Symposia on Child Psychology* (Vol. 7). Hillsdale, NJ: Erlbaum.

Feuerstein, R. (1979). *Dynamic assessment of retarded performers.* Baltimore: University Park Press.

Feuerstein, R. (1980). *Instrumental enrichment.* Baltimore: University Park Press.

Feuerstein, R. (1981). Mediated Learning Experience in the acquisition of kinesics. In B. L. Hoffer & R. N. St. Clair (Eds.), *Developmental kinesics: The emerging paradigm.* Baltimore: University Park Press.

Feuerstein, R. (1987, July). [*Theory and characteristics of Mediated Learning Experience.*] Paper presented at the International Conference on Mediated Learning Experience, Jerusalem.

Feuerstein, R., Haywood, H. C., Rand, Y., Hoffman, M. B., & Jensen, M. R. (no date). *L.P.A.D. Learning Potential Assessment Device manual.* Jerusalem: Hadassah–WIZO–Canada Research Institute.

Feuerstein, R., & Hoffman, M. B. (1982). Intergenerational conflict of rights: Cultural imposition and self-realization. *Viewpoints in Teaching and Learning* (Journal of the School of Education, Indiana University), *58*, 44–63.

Feuerstein, R., Klein, P. S., & Tannenbaum, A. J. (Eds.). (in press). *Mediated Learning Experience (MLE): Theoretical, psychosocial, and learning implications.* London: Freund.

Feuerstein, R., & Rand, Y. (1973-1975). Mediated Learning Experiences: An outline of the proximal etiology for differential development of cognitive functions. In *International understanding: Cultural differences in the development of cognitive processes.* New York: Women in National and International Psychology (L. G. Fein, Chairwoman).

Feuerstein, R., Rand, Y., & Rynders, J. E. (1988). *Don't accept me as I am: Helping "retarded" people to excel.* New York: Plenum.

Finkelstein, N. E., & Ramey, C. T. (1977). Learning to control the environment in infancy. *Child Development, 48,* 806–819.

Flavell, J. H. (1985). *Cognitive development* (2nd ed.). Englewood Cliffs, NJ: Prentice-Hall.

Friedman, S. L., Gordon, M. A., & Ross, M. C. (1986). *Mediation of toddlers' cognitive development by mothers with and without psychiatric diagnosis of depression.* (ERIC Document Reproduction Service No. ED 272 309)

Fry, P. S., & Lupart, J. L. (1987). *Cognitive processes in children's learning: Practical applications in educational practice and classroom management.* Springfield, IL: Charles C Thomas.

Glaser, R. (1981). The future of testing: A research agenda for cognitive psychology and psychometrics. *American Psychologist, 36,* 923–936.

Glazier-Robinson, B. A. (1986). *The relationship between mediated learning and academic achievement.* Unpublished master's thesis, Bryn Mawr College.

Glazier-Robinson, B. A. (1990). *Improving the ability of low SES mothers to provide Mediated Learning Experiences for their four year old children.* Unpublished doctoral dissertation, Bryn Mawr College.

Goldberg, R. J. (1982). Learning in the family context: Research on parents' perceptions of their role as educator of young children. In N. Nir-Janiv, B. Spodek, & D. Steg (Eds.), *Early childhood education: An international perspective.* New York: Plenum.

Gordon, J. E., & Haywood, H. C. (1969). Input deficit in cultured–familial retardates: Effect of stimulus enrichment. *American Journal of Mental Deficiency, 73,* 604–610.

Gottfried, A. W. (1985). The relationships of play materials and parental involvement to young children's development. In C. C. Brown & A. W. Gottfried (Eds.), *The role of toys and parental involvement in children's development*. Skillman, NJ: Johnson & Johnson.

Greenberg, K. H. (1987). *Mediated Learning Experience Observation Analysis System*. Unpublished manuscript, Department of Special Education and Rehabilitation, University of Tennessee.

Greenberg, K. H. (1990). Mediated learning in the classroom. *International Journal of Cognitive Education and Mediated Learning, 1*, 33–44.

Gupta, R. M., & Coxhead, P. (Eds.). (1988). *Cultural diversity and learning efficiency: Recent developments in assessment*. New York: St. Martin's Press.

Guthke, J. (1982). The learning test concept: An alternative to the traditional static intelligence test. *German Journal of Psychology, 6*, 306–324.

Haeussermann, E. (1958). *Developmental potential of preschool children*. New York: Grune & Stratton.

Hamers, J. H. M. (Ed.). (in press). *Dynamic assessment: European contributions*. Amsterdam: Swets & Zeitlinger.

Hamilton, J., & Budoff, M. (1974). *Learning potential among the moderately and severely mentally retarded* (RIEPrint No. 52). Cambridge, MA: Research Institute for Educational Problems.

Haywood, H. C., Filler, J. W., Jr., Shifman, M. A. & Chatalanet, G. (1975). Behavioral assessment in mental retardation. In P. McReynolds (Ed.), *Advances in psychological assessment* (Vol. 3). San Francisco: Jossey-Bass.

Haywood, H. C., & Switzky, H. N. (1974). Children's verbal abstracting: Effects of enriched input, age, and IQ. *American Journal of Mental Deficiency, 78*, 556–565.

Heckhausen, J. (1987). Balancing for weaknesses and challenging developmental potential: A longitudinal study of mother–infant dyads in apprenticeship interactions. *Developmental Psychology, 23*, 762–770.

Hegarty, S. (1979). *Manual for the Test of Children's Learning Ability — individual version* (research ed.). Windsor, England: National Foundation for Educational Research.

Hegarty, S. (1988). Learning ability and psychometric practice. In R. M. Gupta & P. Coxhead (Eds.), *Cultural diversity and learning efficiency: Recent developments in assessment*. New York: St. Martin's Press.

Hess, R. D., Kashiwagi, K., Azuma, H., Price, G. D., & Dickson, W. P. (1980). Maternal expectations for mastery of developmental tasks in Japan and the United States. *International Journal of Psychology, 15*, 259–271.

Hess, R. D., & Shipman, V. C. (1968). Maternal influences upon early learning: The cognitive environments of urban pre-school children. In R. D. Hess & R. M. Baer (Eds.), *Early education: Current theory, research, and action*. Chicago: Aldine.

Hess, R. D., & Shipman, V. C. (1973). Early blocks to children's learning. In R. D. Strom & E. P. Torrance (Eds.), *Education for affective achievement*. Chicago: Rand McNally.

Hitz, R., & Driscoll, R. (1988). Praise or encouragement? New insights into praise: Implications for early childhood teachers. *Young Children, 43,* 6–13.

Huberty, T. J., & Cross, R. W. (1988). Feuerstein's Representational Stencil Design Test: A comparison of two scoring methods. *Journal of Psychoeducational Assessment, 6,* 207–214.

Huberty, T. J., & Koller, J. R. (1984). A test of the learning potential hypothesis with hearing and deaf students. *Journal of Educational Research, 78,* 22–28.

Jensen, M. R., & Feuerstein, R. (1987). The Learning Potential Assessment Device: From philosophy to practice. In C. S. Lidz (Ed.), *Dynamic assessment: An interactional approach to evaluating learning potential.* New York: Guilford Press.

Johnson, J. E., & Martin, C. (1985). Parents' beliefs and home learning environments: Effects on cognitive development. In I. E. Sigel (Ed.), *Parental belief systems.* Hillsdale, NJ: Erlbaum.

Kahn, R. J. (1988). *Manual for observations of Mediated Learning Experiences.* Unpublished manuscript, Family Development Resource Center, St. Joseph College, West Hartford, CT.

Kaniel, S., Tzuriel, D., Feuerstein, R., Ben Shachar, N., & Eitan, T. (1989). *Dynamic assessment: Learning and transfer abilities of Ethiopian immigrants to Israel.* Unpublished manuscript, Bar Ilan University, School of Education, Ramat Gan, Israel.

Katz, M. A., & Buchholz, E. S. (1984). Use of the LPAD for cognitive enrichment of a deaf child. *School Psychology Review, 13,* 99–106.

Kaufman, A. S., & Kaufman, N. L. (1983). *K-ABC. Kaufman Assessment Battery for Children: Administration and scoring manual, and interpretive manual.* Circle Pines, MN: American Guidance Service.

Keane, K. J., & Kretschmer, R. E. (1987). Effect of mediated learning intervention on cognitive task performance with a deaf population. *Journal of Educational Psychology, 79,* 49–53.

Kinsbourne, M., & Caplan, P. J. (1979). *Children's learning and attention problems.* Boston: Little, Brown.

Kirby, E. A., & Grimley, L. K. (1986). *Understanding and treating attention deficit disorder.* Elmsford, NY: Pergamon Press.

Klein, P. S. (1988). Stability and change in interaction of Israeli mothers and infants. *Infant Behavior and Development, 11,* 55–70.

Klein, P. S. (no date). *Criteria for observation of Mediated Learning Experience in infancy and early childhood.* Unpublished manuscript, Bar Ilan University, School of Education, Ramat Gan, Israel.

Klein, P. S., & Feuerstein, R. (1985). Environmental variables and cognitive development: Identification of the potent factors in parent–child interactions. In S. Harel & N. J. Anastasiow (Eds.), *The at-risk infant: Psycho/socio/medical aspects.* Baltimore: Paul H. Brookes.

Klein, P. S., Wieder, S., & Greenspan, S. I. (1987). A theoretical overview and empirical study of Mediated Learning Experience: Prediction of preschool performance from mother–infant interaction patterns. *Infant Mental Health Journal, 8,* 110–129.

Kuczynski, L. (1984). Socialization goals and mother–child interaction: Strategies for long-term and short-term compliance. *Developmental Psychology, 20,* 1061–1073.

Kuczynski, L., Kochanska, G., Radke-Yarrow, M., & Girnius-Brown, O. (1987). A developmental interpretation of young children's noncompliance. *Developmental Psychology, 23,* 799–806.

Levenstein, P. (1979). The parent–child network. In A. Simmons-Martin & S. E. Calvert (Eds.), *Parent–infant intervention: Communication disorders.* New York: Grune & Stratton.

Lewis, M. (1978). The infant and its caregiver: The role of contingency. *Allied Health and Behavioral Sciences, 1,* 469–492.

Lewis, M., & Fox, N. (1980). Predicting cognitive development from assessments in infancy. In B. W. Camp (Ed.), *Advances in behavioral pediatrics* (Vol. 1). Greenwich, CT: JAI Press.

Lewis, M., & Goldberg, S. (1969). Perceptual–cognitive development in infancy: A generalized expectancy model as a function of the mother–infant interaction. *Merrill–Palmer Quarterly, 15,* 81–100.

Lidz, C. S. (Ed.). (1987a). *Dynamic assessment: An interactional approach to evaluating learning potential.* New York: Guilford Press.

Lidz, C. S. (1987b). Cognitive deficiencies revisited. In C. S. Lidz (Ed.), *Dynamic assessment: An interactional approach to evaluating learning potential.* New York: Guilford Press.

Lidz, C. S. (in press-a). MLE components and their roots in theory and research. In R. Feuerstein, P. S. Klein, & A. J. Tannenbaum (Eds.), *Mediated Learning Experience (MLE): Theoretical, psychosocial, and learning implications.* London: Freund.

Lidz, C. S. (in press-b). The status of dynamic assessment training: A national survey of trainers of school psychologists. *Journal of Special Education.*

Lidz, C. S., Bond, L., & Dissinger, L. (1990). Consistency of mother–child interaction using the Mediated Learning Experience (MLE) Scale. *Special Services in the Schools, 6,* 145–165.

Lidz, C. S., & Thomas, C. (1987). The Preschool Learning Assessment Device: Extension of a static approach. In C. S. Lidz (Ed.), *Dynamic assessment: An interactional approach to evaluating learning potential.* New York: Guilford Press.

Luria, A. R. (1966). *Human brain and psychological processes* (B. Haigh, Trans.). New York: Harper & Row.

Luria, A. R. (1973). *The working brain* (B. Haigh, Trans.). New York: Basic Books.

Luther, M., & Wyatt, F. (1990). A comparison of Feuerstein's method of (LPAD) assessment with conventional I.Q. testing on disadvantaged North York high school students. *International Journal of Dynamic Assessment and Instruction, 1,* 49–64.

Maccoby, E., & Martin, J. (1983). Socialization in the context of the family:

Parent–child interaction. In E. M. Hetherington (Vol. Ed.), *Handbook of child psychology* (4th ed.): *Vol. 4. Socialization, personality, and social development.* New York: Wiley.

Maccoby, E., Snow, M. E., & Jacklin, C. N. (1984). Children's dispositions and mother–child interaction at 12 and 18 months: A short-term longitudinal study. *Developmental Psychology, 20,* 459–472.

MacPhee, D. (1981). *Manual: Knowledge of Infant Development Inventory.* Unpublished manuscript, University of North Carolina.

McClelland, D. C. (1973). Testing for competence rather than for "intelligence." *American Psychologist, 28,* 1–14.

McGillicuddy-DeLisi, A. V. (1985). The relationship between parental beliefs and children's cognitive level. In I. E. Sigel (Ed.), *Parental belief systems.* Hillsdale, NJ: Erlbaum.

McGillicuddy-DeLisi, A. V., Sigel, I. E., & Johnson, J. E. (1979). The family as a system of mutual influences: Parental beliefs, distancing behaviors and children's representational thinking. In M. Lewis & L. A. Rosenblum (Eds.), *The child and its family.* New York: Plenum.

Mearig, J. S. (1987). Assessing the learning potential of kindergarten and primary-age children. In C. S. Lidz (Ed.), *Dynamic assessment: An interactional approach to evaluating learning potential.* New York: Guilford Press.

Miller, S. A. (1988). Parents' beliefs about children's cognitive development. *Child Development, 59,* 259–285.

Minick, N. (1987). Implications of Vygotsky's theories for dynamic assessment. In C. S. Lidz (Ed.), *Dynamic assessment: An interactional approach to evaluating learning potential.* New York: Guilford Press.

Missiuna, C. (1986). *Dynamic assessment of preschool children with special needs: Comparison of mediation and instruction.* Unpublished master's thesis, University of Calgary.

Naglieri, J. A. (1989). A cognitive processing theory for the measurement of intelligence. *Educational Psychologist, 24,* 185–206.

Naglieri, J. A., & Das, J. P. (1988). Planning–arousal–simultaneous–successive (PASS): A model for assessment. *Journal of School Psychology, 26,* 35–48.

Naglieri, J. A., Das, J. P., & Jarman, R. F. (1990). Planning, attention, simultaneous, and successive cognitive processes as a model for assessment. *School Psychology Review, 19,* 423–442.

Norman, D. A. (1976). *Memory and attention: An introduction to human information processing.* New York: Wiley.

Norman-Jackson, J. (1982). Family interactions, language development, and primary reading achievement of black children in families of low income. *Child Development, 53,* 349–358.

Olson, S. L., Bates, J. E., & Bayles, K. (1984). Mother–infant interaction and the development of individual differences in children's cognitive competence. *Developmental Psychology, 20,* 166–170.

Ortar, G. R. (1959). Improving test validity with coaching. *Educational Research, 2,* 137–142.

Palincsar, A. S., & Brown, A. L. (1984). Reciprocal teaching of comprehension-fostering and monitoring activities. *Cognition and Instruction, 1,* 117–175.

Paour, J. (in press). Induction of logic structures in the mentally retarded: An assessment and intervention instrument. In H. C. Haywood & D. Tzuriel (Eds.), *Interactive assessment.* New York: Springer.

Penrose, L. S. (1934). *Mental defects.* New York: Farrar & Rinehart.

Popoff-Walker, L. E. (1982). IQ, SES, adaptive behavior, and performance on a learning potential measure. *Journal of School Psychology, 20,* 222–231.

Pratt, M. W., Kerig, P., Cowan, P. A., & Cowan, C. P. (1988). Mothers and fathers teaching 3-year-olds: Authoritative parenting and adult scaffolding. *Developmental Psychology, 24,* 832–839.

Ramey, C. T., Farran, D. C., & Campbell, F. A. (1979). Predicting IQ from mother–child interactions. *Child Development, 50,* 804–814.

Rand, Y., & Kaniel, S. (1987). Group administration of the LPAD. In C. S. Lidz (Ed.), *Dynamic assessment: An interactional approach to evaluating learning potential.* New York: Guilford Press.

Ratner, H. (1980). The role of social context in memory development. In M. Perlmutter (Ed.), *New directions for child development: No. 10. Children's memory.* San Francisco: Jossey-Bass.

Reinharth, B. M. (1989). *Cognitive modifiability in developmentally delayed children.* Unpublished doctoral dissertation, Yeshiva University.

Rocissano, L., & Yatchmink, Y. (1983). Language skill and interactive patterns in prematurely born toddlers. *Child Development, 54,* 1229–1241.

Rohwer, W. D., Jr. (1971). Learning, race, and school success. *Review of Educational Research, 41,* 191–210.

Rohwer, W. D., Jr., & Ammon, M. S. (1971). Elaboration training and paired-associate learning efficiency in children. *Journal of Educational Psychology, 62,* 376–383.

Rosenfield, S. (1987). *Instructional consultation.* Hillsdale, NJ: Erlbaum.

Rutter, M. (1990). Commentary: Some focus and process considerations regarding effects of parental depression on children. *Developmental Psychology, 26,* 60–67.

Samuels, M., Tzuriel, D., & Malloy-Miller, T. (1989). Dynamic assessment of children with learning difficulties. In R. Brown & M. Chazan (Eds.), *Emotional and allied issues in the field of disability.* Calgary: Detselig Press.

Schucman, H. (1960). Evaluating the educability of the severely mentally retarded child. *Psychological Monographs, 74*(14, Whole No. 501).

Scrofani, P. J., Suziedelis, A., & Shore, M. F. (1973). Conceptual ability in black and white children of different social classes: An experimental test of Jensen's hypothesis. *American Journal of Orthopsychiatry, 43,* 541–553.

Sewell, T. E. (1979). Intelligence and learning tasks as predictors of scholastic achievement in black and white first-grade children. *Journal of School Psychology, 17,* 325–332.

Sewell, T. E., & Severson, R. A. (1974). Learning ability and intelligence as cognitive predictors of achievement in first-grade black children. *Journal of Educational Psychology, 66,* 948–955.

Shapiro, E. S. (1989). *Academic skills problems: Direct assessment and intervention.* New York: Guilford Press.

Shinn, M. R. (Ed.). (1989). *Curriculum-based measurement: Assessing special children.* New York: Guilford Press.

Sigel, I. E. (1986). Early social experience and the development of representational competence. In W. Fowler (Ed.), *New directions for child development: No. 32. Early experience and the development of competence.* San Francisco: Jossey-Bass.

Sigel, I. E., & McGillicuddy-DeLisi, A. V. (1984). Parents as teachers of their children: A distancing behavior model. In A. D. Pelligrini & T. D. Yawkey (Eds.), *The development of oral and written language in social contexts.* Norwood, NJ: Ablex.

Skuy, M. S., Archer, M., & Roth, I. (1987). Use of the Learning Potential Assessment Device in assessment and remediation of a learning problem. *South African Journal of Education, 7,* 53–58.

Skuy, M., Kaniel, S., & Tzuriel, D. (1988). Dynamic assessment of intellectually superior Israeli children in a low socioeconomic status community. *Gifted Education International, 5,* 90–96.

Slade, A. (1987). A longitudinal study of maternal involvement and symbolic play during the toddler period. *Child Development, 58,* 367–375.

Speece, D. L., Cooper, D. H., & Kibler, J. M. (1989). Dynamic assessment, individual differences, and academic achievement. In P. L. Ackerman, R. J. Sternberg, & R. Glaser (Eds.), *Learning and individual differences: Advances in theory and research.* New York: W. H. Freeman.

Stern, D. (1984). Affect attunement. In J. Call, E. Golenson, & R. Tyson (Eds.), *Frontiers of infant psychiatry* (Vol. 11). New York: Basic Books.

Stern, G. G., Caldwell, B. M., Hersher, L., Lipton, E. L., & Richmond, J. B. (1969). A factor-analytic study of the mother–infant dyad. *Child Development, 40,* 163–181.

Streissguth, A. P., & Bee, H. L. (1971). Mother–child interactions and cognitive development in children. *Young Children, 27,* 154–173.

Symons, S. E., & Vye, N. J. (1986). *Instructional components of mediational dynamic assessment* (Alternative Assessments of Handicapped Children, Technical Report No. 6). Nashville, TN: John F. Kennedy Center for Research on Education and Human Development, Vanderbilt University.

Thomas, C. (1986). *The effects of mediation on the performance of disadvantaged preschool children on two cognitive tasks.* Unpublished doctoral dissertation, Bryn Mawr College.

Tomasello, M., & Farrar, M. (1986). Joint attention and early language. *Child Development, 57,* 1454–1463.

Tyler, L. E. (1976). The intelligence we test: An evolving concept. In L. B. Resnick (Ed.), *The nature of intelligence.* Hillsdale, NJ: Erlbaum.

Tzuriel, D. (1989). Inferential thinking modifiability in young socially disadvantaged and advantaged children. *International Journal of Dynamic Assessment and Instruction, 1,* 65–80.

Tzuriel, D., & Eran, Z. (1989, August 6–8). *Inferential cognitive modifiability of kibbutz young children as a function of mother–child MLE interaction.* Paper presented at the Second International Conference on Mediated Learning Experience, Knoxville, TN.

Tzuriel, D., & Klein, P. S. (1985). Analogical thinking modifiability in disadvantaged, regular, special education, and mentally retarded children. *Journal of Abnormal Child Psychology, 13,* 539–552.

Tzuriel, D., & Klein, P. S. (1986). *The Frame Test of Cognitive Modifiability Manual.* Ramat Gan, Israel: Bar Ilan University.

Tzuriel, D., & Klein, P. S. (1987). Assessing the young child: Children's analogical thinking modifiability. In C. S. Lidz (Ed.), *Dynamic assessment: An interactional approach to evaluating learning potential.* New York: Guilford Press.

Tzuriel, D., & Klein, P. S. (no date). *The dynamic method: A different approach to decision making about cognitive modifiability of young children.* Unpublished manuscript, Bar Ilan University, School of Education, Ramat Gan, Israel.

Vaught, S. R., & Haywood, H. C. (1989, August 6–8). *Interjudge agreement in dynamic assessment: Two instruments from the Learning Potential Assessment Device.* Paper presented at the Second International Conference on Mediated Learning Experience, Knoxville, TN.

Vietze, P. M., & Anderson, B. J. (1981). Styles of parent–child interaction. In M. J. Begab, H. C. Haywood, & H. L. Garber (Eds.), *Psychosocial influences in retarded performance* (Vol. 1). Baltimore: University Park Press.

Vye, N. J., Burns, M. S., Delclos, V. R., & Bransford, J. D. (1987). A comprehensive approach to assessing intellectually handicapped children. In C. S. Lidz (Ed.), *Dynamic assessment: An interactional approach to evaluating learning potential.* New York: Guilford Press.

Vygotsky, L. S. (1978). *Mind in society: The development of higher psychological processes* (M. Cole, V. John-Steiner, S. Scribner, & E. Souberman, Eds.). Cambridge, MA: Harvard University Press.

Vygotsky, L. S. (1986). *Thought and language* (A. Kozulin, Trans.). Cambridge, MA: MIT Press.

Watts, W. J. (1985). An error analysis on the Raven's using Feuerstein's deficient cognitive functions. *Alberta Journal of Educational Research, 31,* 41–53.

Weinstein, C. E., & Mayer, R. E. (1986). The teaching of learning strategies. In M. C. Wittrock (Ed.), *Handbook of research on teaching* (3rd ed.). New York: Macmillan.

Wertsch, J. V. (1979). From social interaction to higher psychological processes: A clarification and application of Vygotsky's theory. *Human Development, 22,* 1–22.

Wittrock, M. C. (1986). Students' thought processes. In M. C. Wittrock (Ed.), *Handbook of research on teaching* (3rd ed.). New York: Macmillan.

Wood, D. (1980). Teaching the young child: Some relationships between social interaction, language, and thought. In D. R. Olson (Ed.), *The social foundation of language and thought.* New York: Norton.

Wood, D., Bruner, J., & Ross, G. (1976). The role of tutoring in problem-solving. *Journal of Child Psychology and Psychiatry, 17,* 89–100.

Wurtz, R., Sewell, T., & Manni, J. L. (1985). The relationship of Estimated Learning Potential to performance on a learning task and achievement. *Psychology in the Schools, 22,* 293–302.

Yarrow, L. J., Morgan, G. A., Jennings, K. D., Harmon, R. J., & Gaiter, J. L. (1982). Infants' persistence at tasks: Relationship to cognitive functioning and early experience. *Infant Behavior and Development, 5,* 131–141.

Yarrow, L. J., Rubenstein, J. L., Pederson, F. R., & Jankowski, J. J. (1972). Dimensions of early stimulation and their differential effects on infant development. *Merrill-Palmer Quarterly, 18,* 205–218.

Zaslow, M. J., Rabinovich, B. A., Suwalsky, J. T. D., & Klein, A. P. (1988). The role of social context in the prediction of secure and insecure/avoidant infant–mother attachment. *Journal of Applied Developmental Psychology, 9,* 287–299.

Index